INTERVENTIONAL CARDIOLOGY CLINICS

www.interventional.theclinics.com

Editor-in-Chief

MATTHEW J. PRICE

Intravascular Imaging: OCT and IVUS

July 2015 • Volume 4 • Number 3

Editor

MATTHEW J. PRICE

ELSEVIER

1600 John F. Kennedy Boulevard • Suite 1800 • Philadelphia, Pennsylvania, 19103-2899

http://www.theclinics.com

INTERVENTIONAL CARDIOLOGY CLINICS Volume 4, Number 3
July 2015 ISSN 2211-7458, ISBN-13: 978-0-323-39103-0

Editor: Adrianne Brigido
Developmental Editor: Barbara Cohen-Kligerman

Interventional Cardiology Clinics (ISSN 2211-7458) is published quarterly by Elsevier Inc., 360 Park Avenue South, New York, NY 10010-1710. Months of issue are January, April, July, and October. Subscription prices are USD 195 per year for US individuals, USD 305 for US institutions, USD 130 per year for US students, USD 230 per year for Canadian individuals, USD 375 for Canadian institutions, USD 150 per year for Canadian students, USD 295 per year for international individuals, USD 375 for international institutions, and USD 150 per year for international students. To receive student/resident rate, orders must be accompanied by name of affiliated institution, date of term, and the *signature* of program/residency coordinator on institution letterhead. Orders will be billed at individual rate until proof of status is received. Foreign air speed delivery is included in all *Clinics* subscription prices. All prices are subject to change without notice. **POSTMASTER:** Send address changes to *Interventional Cardiology Clinics*, Elsevier Health Sciences Division, Subscription Customer Service, 3251 Riverport Lane, Maryland Heights, MO 63043. **Customer Service: Telephone: 1-800-654-2452** (U.S. and Canada); **1-314-447-8871** (outside U.S. and Canada). **Fax: 1-314-447-8029. E-mail: journalscustomerservice-usa@elsevier.com (for print support);** journalsonlinesupport-usa@elsevier.com **(for online support)**.

Reprints. For copies of 100 or more of articles in this publication, please contact the Commercial Reprints Department, Elsevier Inc., 360 Park Avenue South, New York, NY 10010-1710. Tel.: 212-633-3874; Fax: 212-633-3820; E-mail: reprints@elsevier.com.

CONTRIBUTORS

EDITOR-IN-CHIEF

MATTHEW J. PRICE, MD
Assistant Professor, Scripps Translational
Science Institute; Director of the Cardiac
Catheterization Laboratory, Scripps
Green Hospital, La Jolla, California

EDITOR

MATTHEW J. PRICE, MD
Assistant Professor, Scripps Translational
Science Institute; Director of the Cardiac
Catheterization Laboratory, Scripps
Green Hospital, La Jolla, California

AUTHORS

TOM ADRIAENSSENS, MD, PhD
Department of Cardiovascular Sciences,
Katholieke Universiteit Leuven; Departments
of Cardiovascular Diseases and Cardiovascular
Medicine, University Hospitals Leuven,
Leuven, Belgium

JUNG-MIN AHN, MD
Division of Cardiology, Asan Medical Center,
University of Ulsan College of Medicine,
Seoul, Korea

BENEDETTA BELLANDI, MD
Department of Cardiology, Careggi Hospital,
Florence, Italy

CHIARA BERNELLI, MD
Interventional Cardiology Unit, Azienda
Ospedaliera Papa Giovanni XXIII, Bergamo,
Italy

TAMARA GARCIA CAMARERO, MD
Interventional Cardiology Department,
Unidad de Cardiología Intervencionista,
Hospital Universitario Marques de Valdecilla,
Santander, Spain

CARLOS M. CAMPOS, MD
Department of Interventional Cardiology,
Thoraxcenter, Erasmus University Medical
Centre, Rotterdam, The Netherlands;
Department of Interventional Cardiology
Heart Institute (InCor), University of São Paulo
Medical School, Sao Paulo, Brazil

JOSE M. DE LA TORRE HERNANDEZ,
MD, PhD, FESC
Interventional Cardiology Department,
Unidad de Cardiología Intervencionista,
Hospital Universitario Marques de
Valdecilla, Santander, Spain

LIM ENG, MD
Division of Cardiology, Vancouver General
Hospital, University of British Columbia,
Vancouver, British Columbia, Canada

CHRISTOPHER FRANCO, MD, PhD
Division of Cardiology, Vancouver General
Hospital, University of British Columbia,
Vancouver, British Columbia, Canada

HECTOR M. GARCIA-GARCIA, MD, PhD
Department of Interventional Cardiology,
Thoraxcenter, Erasmus University Medical
Centre; Medical Affairs, Cardialysis,
Rotterdam, The Netherlands

GIULIO GUAGLIUMI, MD, FESC
Interventional Cardiology Unit, Azienda
Ospedaliera Papa Giovanni XXIII,
Bergamo, Italy

MYEONG-KI HONG, MD, PhD
Division of Cardiology, Severance Cardiovascular
Hospital, Yonsei University College of Medicine,
Yonsei University Health System; Cardiovascular
Institute, Yonsei University College of Medicine;
Severance Biomedical Science Institute, Yonsei
University College of Medicine, Seodaemun-gu,
Seoul, Korea

IK-KYUNG JANG, MD, PhD
Professor of Medicine, Cardiology Division, Massachusetts General Hospital, Harvard Medical School, Boston, Massachusetts; Division of Cardiology, Kyung Hee University, Seoul, Korea

ARABINDRA B. KATWAL, MBBS
Division of Cardiology, Department of Medicine, Stritch School of Medicine, Loyola University Medical Center, Maywood, Illinois

SEUNG-YUL LEE, MD
Division of Cardiology, Sanbon Hospital, Wonkwang University College of Medicine, Gunpo, Gyeonggido, Korea

JOHN J. LOPEZ, MD
Division of Cardiology, Department of Medicine, Stritch School of Medicine, Loyola University Medical Center, Maywood, Illinois

AKIKO MAEHARA, MD
Department of Medicine, Columbia University Medical Center; Clinical Trials Center, Cardiovascular Research Foundation, New York, New York

MITSUAKI MATSUMURA, BS
Clinical Trials Center, Cardiovascular Research Foundation, New York, New York

ALESSIO MATTESINI, MD
Department of Cardiology, Careggi Hospital, Florence, Italy

GARY S. MINTZ, MD
Clinical Trials Center, Cardiovascular Research Foundation, New York, New York

SHIMPEI NAKATANI, MD
Department of Interventional Cardiology, Thoraxcenter, Erasmus University Medical Centre, Rotterdam, The Netherlands

DANIEL S. ONG, MD
Clinical and Research Fellow in Cardiovascular Medicine, Cardiology Division, Massachusetts General Hospital, Harvard Medical School, Boston, Massachusetts

YOSHINOBU ONUMA, MD, PhD
Department of Interventional Cardiology, Thoraxcenter, Erasmus University Medical Centre, Rotterdam, The Netherlands

SEUNG-JUNG PARK, MD, PhD
Professor of Medicine, Division of Cardiology, Asan Medical Center, University of Ulsan College of Medicine, Seoul, Korea

GUIDO PARODI, MD, PhD, FESC
Department of Cardiology, Careggi Hospital, Florence, Italy

JACQUELINE SAW, MD, FRCPC, FACC
Clinical Associate Professor, Division of Cardiology, Vancouver General Hospital, University of British Columbia, Vancouver, British Columbia, Canada

PATRICK W. SERRUYS, MD, PhD
Department of Interventional Cardiology, Thoraxcenter, Erasmus University Medical Centre, Rotterdam, The Netherlands; International Centre for Circulatory Health, National Heart and Lung Institute, Imperial College London, London, United Kingdom

VASILE SIRBU, MD
Interventional Cardiology Unit, Azienda Ospedaliera Papa Giovanni XXIII, Bergamo, Italy

PANNIPA SUWANNASOM, MD
Department of Interventional Cardiology, Thoraxcenter, Erasmus University Medical Centre, Rotterdam, The Netherlands

GIOVANNI J. UGHI, PhD
Department of Cardiovascular Sciences, Katholieke Universiteit Leuven; Department of Cardiovascular Diseases, University Hospitals Leuven, Leuven, Belgium

SERAFINA VALENTE, MD
Department of Cardiology, Careggi Hospital, Florence, Italy

CONTENTS

Optical coherence tomography (OCT) is an intravascular imaging modality that enables high-resolution cross-sectional imaging of coronary arteries in vivo. With resolution that is a 10-fold improvement compared with intravascular ultrasonography, OCT can facilitate detailed plaque characterization. This article introduces the basic principles of OCT image acquisition and interpretation. Qualitative analysis entails the evaluation of plaque morphology, including features associated with plaque vulnerability to rupture. Quantitative analysis and recognition of OCT image artifacts are also discussed.

Optical coherence tomography (OCT) is an intravascular imaging technology analogous to intravascular ultrasound, using near-infrared light rather than ultrasound, thereby providing higher-resolution images. This review provides a practical guide to OCT imaging, with a particular emphasis on the techniques and approaches to optimize image acquisition, improve the evaluation of coronary lesions, and guide the strategies for percutaneous coronary intervention.

 Videos of OCT to diagnose nonatherosclerotic disease and OCT pull back accompany this article

Although coronary angiography is used to confirm or exclude coronary artery disease, assess lesion severity, and help determine percutaneous coronary interventions (PCI), it has clear limitations. Intravascular imaging has emerged to guide more precise PCI. Frequency domain optical coherence tomography (OCT) has gained attention for accurate planning and guidance of complex PCI. High-speed OCT image acquisition enables prompt vessel assessment in stable and unstable patients. The high-resolution images provide precise tissue characterization and a reliable quantitative assessment of the coronary pathology. Immediately after stent implantation, OCT allows accurate evaluation of stent expansion and symmetry. Real-time angio-OCT co-registration integrates OCT into the PCI workflow for accurate decision-making.

Optical coherence tomography evaluation of poststent results includes the following: (1) stent expansion as the absolute minimum stent area (MSA) ratio by comparing the MSA with the proximal and distal reference lumen areas or mean stent area defined as the total stent volume divided by the analyzed stent length; (2) stent strut malapposition defined when the distance from the center of the blooming artifact and the surface of plaque is greater than the sum of stent thickness and polymer thickness; (3) tissue protrusion through the stent struts; (4) semiquantitative residual thrombus evaluation; and (5) stent edge dissection.

Stent thrombosis (ST) is a rare complication of percutaneous coronary interventions (PCI), especially with drug-eluting stents. ST presents as acute myocardial infarction requiring emergent repeat PCI; optimal reperfusion occurs in two-thirds of patients. As a result, ST has been associated with a high mortality rate and a high rate of recurrent thrombosis. We discuss the use of optical coherence tomography (OCT) for the diagnosis and evaluation of ST. OCT-guided ST management seems a feasible, safe, and appropriate approach. Intracoronary imaging is able to assess the efficacy of coronary thrombus removal procedures and detect the prevalent stent-related factor that caused ST.

Spontaneous coronary artery dissection (SCAD) is an infrequent condition that has been underdiagnosed and misdiagnosed. The use of intracoronary imaging with intravascular ultrasound or optical coherence tomography enables the accurate diagnosis of this challenging condition. Diagnostic and management algorithms have been proposed to improve the diagnosis and therapeutic stratification of SCAD. Optical coherence tomography has superior spatial resolution compared to intravascular ultrasound, and is instrumental in the diagnosis of SCAD cases where angiographic findings are ambiguous for confirming SCAD. Understanding the role and appropriate and careful use of this technology is expected to improve the diagnosis of SCAD, and also improve outcomes with percutaneous coronary intervention, when clinically indicated.

Based on high resolution, optical coherence tomography (OCT) has provided novel insights into the pathophysiology of neointimal growth after drug-eluting stent (DES) implantation. Strut coverage, an indirect marker of neointimal healing, is associated with DES type and malapposition. Use of a newer-generation DES improves strut coverage, and subsequently reduces the development of stent thrombosis. Substantial malapposition delays strut coverage and may play a role as substrate for stent thrombosis. Neoatherosclerosis contributes to progressive neointimal hyperplasia and provides the vulnerability causing acute coronary syndrome or stent thrombosis. Accordingly, novel strategies using OCT are anticipated for the treatment of ischemic heart disease.

The analysis of bioresorbable scaffolds (BRSs) by optical coherence tomography (OCT) requires a dedicated methodology, as the polymeric scaffold has a distinct appearance and undergoes dynamic structural changes with time. The high resolution of OCT allows for the detailed assessment of scaffold implantation, rupture, discontinuity, and strut integration. OCT does not provide reliable information on the extent of scaffold degradation, as it cannot differentiate between polylactide polymer and the provisional matrix of proteoglycan formed by connective tissue. Three-dimensional OCT reconstruction can aid in the evaluation of BRS in special scenarios such as overlapping scaffold segments and bifurcations.

Intravascular optical coherence tomography (OCT) is capable of acquiring 3-dimensional (3D) data on coronary arteries, allowing for the assessment of plaques, stents, thrombus, side branches, and other relevant structures in a 3D fashion. Given that state-of-the-art OCT systems acquire images at a very high frame rate (up to 200 frames per second), typically a very large number of images per pullback (ie, 500 or more) need to be analyzed. The manual assessment of stents, plaques, and other structures is time-consuming, cumbersome, and inefficient and thus not suitable for on-line analysis during percutaneous coronary intervention procedures.

The limitations of angiography for assessment of coronary artery disease are well-known but are more evident and relevant in the left main coronary artery (LMCA) segment given the amount of myocardium this vessel subtends and the risks associated with the presence of atherosclerosis and subsequent intervention. Intravascular ultrasound (IVUS) characterizes the severity of luminal narrowing, plaque morphology, and plaque extension into the distal bifurcation. Once the indication for percutaneous intervention (PCI) is established, information provided by IVUS is crucial for planning treatment and optimizing results. IVUS-guided PCI with drug-eluting stents improves clinical outcomes, particularly in patients with distal left main disease.

Intravascular ultrasound (IVUS) has provided valuable information on cross-sectional coronary vascular structure and has played a key role in contemporary stent-based percutaneous coronary interventions (PCI). It accurately assesses coronary anatomy, assists in the selection of treatment strategy, and helps to optimize stenting outcomes. IVUS-guided PCI for drug-eluting stent implantation seems to be associated with a significantly reduced risk of death, myocardial infarction, target lesion revascularization, and stent thrombosis.

INTRAVASCULAR IMAGING: OCT AND IVUS

THE CLINICS ARE NOW AVAILABLE ONLINE!
Access your subscription at:
www.theclinics.com

Fundamentals of Optical Coherence Tomography
Image Acquisition and Interpretation

Daniel S. Ong, MD[a], Ik-Kyung Jang, MD, PhD[a,b,*]

KEYWORDS

- Optical coherence tomography • Intracoronary imaging • Image interpretation • Vulnerable plaque

---

KEY POINTS

- Optical coherence tomography (OCT) is a catheter-based modality that enables in vivo imaging of coronary arteries with 10-fold improved resolution compared with intravascular ultrasonography.
- The high resolution of OCT imaging allows it to serve as an "optical biopsy," facilitating detailed plaque characterization and evaluation of features associated with plaque vulnerability.
- Limitations of OCT include its limited depth of penetration and the need to create a blood-free field during imaging.
- Improvements in image acquisition speed have enabled the translation of OCT from the research setting to clinical practice, and studies are now underway to evaluate OCT-guided decision making.

INTRODUCTION

Optical coherence tomography (OCT) is an emerging catheter-based intravascular imaging modality that enables high-resolution cross-sectional imaging of coronary arteries in vivo. By measuring the magnitude and time delay of backscattered light waves in a manner analogous to the use of sound waves in intravascular ultrasonography (IVUS) imaging, OCT produces images with 10-times improved resolution compared with IVUS.[1] OCT is widely used in ophthalmology for evaluation of the retina,[2] and its application to vascular imaging has enabled detailed plaque characterization,[3] opening up significant opportunities for application in both research and clinical settings.[4] This article introduces the basic principles of OCT image acquisition and interpretation for coronary arteries.

PRINCIPLES OF OPTICAL COHERENCE TOMOGRAPHY IMAGE ACQUISITION

The first generation of OCT platforms used a time domain (TD) detection system in which light from a broadband source with wavelengths centered on 1300 nm was directed at the tissue of interest. Determination of imaged tissue depth required a reference mirror to be moved back and forth, significantly limiting the speed of image acquisition.[3] The second generation of OCT platforms uses a technology called Fourier or frequency domain (FD) detection in which a monochromatic source emits light sweeping across a range of wavelengths between 1250

Disclosures: Dr I.-K. Jang reports receiving a research grant and honorarium from St. Jude Medical and research grants from Medtronic and Boston Scientific Corp.
[a] Cardiology Division, Massachusetts General Hospital, Harvard Medical School, 55 Fruit Street, Boston, MA 02114, USA; [b] Division of Cardiology, Kyung Hee University, 26 Kyungheedae-ro, Dongdaemun-gu, Seoul 130-701, Korea
* Corresponding author. Cardiovascular Division, Massachusetts General Hospital, Harvard Medical School, GRB 800, 55 Fruit Street, Boston, MA 02114.
E-mail address: ijang@mgh.harvard.edu

and 1350 nm. Reflected light from various tissue depths can therefore be detected simultaneously, facilitating significantly faster image acquisition (Fig. 1).[5] The technical specifications of IVUS, TD-OCT, and FD-OCT imaging are compared in Table 1.

An important consideration in the use of OCT as an intravascular imaging modality is that blood must be cleared or flushed from the vessel lumen, because the backscatter of light by red blood cells precludes OCT imaging through a blood field.[6] Initially, blood clearance was accomplished using the occlusion technique, in which an occlusive balloon was inflated proximally to stop coronary blood flow, and saline or Ringer lactate was infused downstream to clear the vessel of blood during pullback imaging. Limitations to this technique include ischemia during balloon occlusion, potential damage to the vessel at the site of balloon occlusion, the need for multiple catheter exchanges, and the inability to image ostial lesions.[7] In addition, vessel dimensions measured on OCT images obtained with the occlusion

technique may be artificially small because of reduced intracoronary pressure downstream from the occlusion balloon.[8,9] Improvements in image acquisition speed have enabled the use of a nonocclusion technique to clear blood from the vessel. In this technique, pullback imaging is performed with simultaneous infusion of saline or contrast through the guide catheter.[10]

At present, FD-OCT imaging is most commonly performed using the C7XR system (LightLab Imaging Inc/St. Jude Medical, Westford, MA). With this system, pullback imaging of up to 54 mm in length can be acquired in 2.7 seconds with 10 to 15 μm axial and 20 to 40 μm lateral resolution.[11] Newer FD-OCT systems such as the ILUMIEN and ILUMIEN OPTIS OCT Intravascular Imaging Systems (St. Jude Medical, St. Paul, MN) have recently become commercially available and are replacing the C7XR system, because they offer additional features to facilitate improved image acquisition and real-time interpretation, including faster pullback speed, longer pullback length, automated measurements,

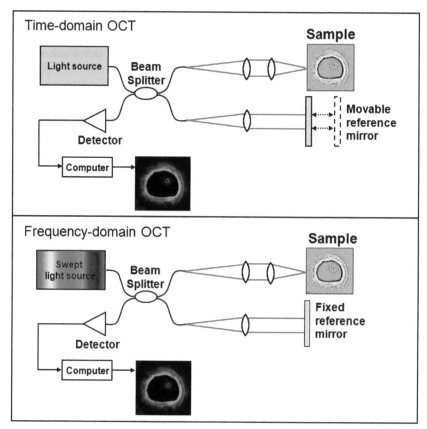

Fig. 1. TD-OCT and FD-OCT. (*From* Soeda T, Uemura S, Saito Y, et al. Optical coherence tomography and coronary plaque characterization. J Jpn Coron Assoc 2013;19(4):309; with permission.)

Table 1
Comparison of IVUS, TD-OCT, and FD-OCT

	IVUS	TD-OCT	FD-OCT
Wavelength (μm)	35–80	1.3	1.3
Axial resolution (μm)	100	15	15
Lateral resolution (μm)	200	90	20–40
Lines (axial scans/frame)	256	200	500
Frame rate (frames/s)	30	16–20	100
Pullback speed (mm/s)	0.5–1.0	1–3	20
Maximum scan diameter (mm)	15–20	6.8	9.7
Tissue penetration (mm)	10	1.0–2.5	2.0–3.5

Data from Lowe HC, Narula J, Fujimoto JG, et al. Intracoronary optical diagnostics current status, limitations, and potential. JACC Cardiovasc Interv 2011;4(12):1259; and Jang IK. Optical coherence tomography or intravascular ultrasound? JACC Cardiovasc Interv 2011;4:493.

three-dimensional image reconstruction, and combined wireless fractional flow reserve measurement capability.

The technique and best practices for performing intracoronary OCT imaging are beyond the scope of this article and are reviewed separately in this issue by Lopez and colleagues.

OPTICAL COHERENCE TOMOGRAPHY IMAGE INTERPRETATION: QUALITATIVE ANALYSIS

OCT imaging offers several unique advantages compared with other intracoronary imaging modalities.[12] Most notably, the high resolution of OCT images enables detailed tissue characterization and plaque analysis, providing an "optical biopsy" in real time.[3] Multiple markers of plaque vulnerability that have been identified on pathology studies have previously been unidentifiable by intravascular imaging because of the limited resolution of IVUS. With OCT, fibrous cap thickness can be accurately measured for the identification of thin-cap fibroatheroma,[6] and other features associated with plaque vulnerability, such as microchannels,[13] macrophages,[14] and cholesterol crystals,[15] can be readily identified.

In contrast with IVUS imaging, which has a depth of penetration of up to 10 mm, OCT imaging is limited by a penetration depth of only 2 to 3 mm.[16] Although this limitation may preclude the use of OCT for accurate measurement of total lipid pool, calculation of plaque burden, or evaluation of vessel remodeling, it has been noted that most relevant features of plaque vulnerability are primarily located in the most superficial 500 μm of the luminal surface (**Table 2**).[6]

Normal Coronary Artery

Recent publications have sought to standardize the methods and nomenclature used in the analysis of OCT images.[7,17–19] The OCT appearance of different structures and tissue components can most easily be described based on their reflectivity (brightness), attenuation, and overall pattern. The

Table 2
Comparison of IVUS and OCT for plaque characterization and stent assessment

	IVUS	OCT
Detection of fibrous cap	–	+++
Detection of lipid	++	+++
Detection of calcium	+++	++
Detection of thrombus	+	++
Evaluation of plaque vulnerability[a]	+	++
Evaluation of plaque burden and remodeling index	+++	–
Post-PCI stent evaluation[b]	++	+++
Late stent follow-up[c]	+	+++

Abbreviation: PCI, percutaneous coronary intervention.
[a] Features associated with plaque vulnerability include thin fibrous caps, large lipid cores, microchannels, macrophage infiltration, superficial spotty calcification, and cholesterol crystals.
[b] Post-PCI stent evaluation includes assessment of stent underexpansion, malapposition, tissue protrusion, and edge dissection.
[c] Late stent follow-up includes evaluation of stent strut coverage, degree of neointimal hyperplasia, malapposition, and neoatherosclerosis.
Data from Jang IK. Optical coherence tomography or intravascular ultrasound? JACC Cardiovasc Interv 2011;4:493.

normal coronary arterial wall appears on OCT as a 3-layered structure composed of an intima, media, and adventitia (Fig. 2). The intima and adventitia appear as bright signal-rich (high-reflectivity) layers, whereas the intervening media appears as a darker signal-poor (low-reflectivity) layer.[6] Although the internal and external elastic lamina that bound the media are below the resolution of OCT and cannot be directly visualized; their location is demarcated by the transition from the signal-rich intima to the signal-poor media and from the signal-poor media to the signal-rich adventitia.

Plaque Characterization

In the presence of atherosclerotic plaque, the 3-layered structure of the normal coronary arterial wall is lost, and the lumen may appear narrowed.[6] Plaques can be categorized by their tissue composition, and the OCT appearance of fibrous, lipid-rich, and calcific plaques has been validated against corresponding histology samples.[6,20,21] Fibrous tissue appears on OCT imaging as a homogeneous area of high reflectivity with low signal attenuation (Fig. 3A). Lipid appears as a homogeneous area of low reflectivity with high signal attenuation that may limit the visualization of deeper structures (see Fig. 3B). Calcium appears as a heterogeneous area of either high or low reflectivity with low signal attenuation and most notably a sharp demarcating border (see Fig. 3C).[6,20] In practice, distinguishing calcium from deep lipid pools can

be challenging,[22] because it is difficult to assess the degree of signal attenuation from structures that are already deep on the OCT image; in these situations, the sharp border delineating calcium deposits can be particularly useful in differentiating it from lipid.[22] Heterogeneity in tissue composition within a single lesion may also contribute to difficulty in categorizing plaques as fibrous, lipid-rich, or calcific.[20,22]

Thrombus is readily identified by OCT as a protruding mass attached to the arterial wall; for image analysis, a measured dimension threshold of greater than or equal to 250 μm has been used to minimize inclusion of small thrombi caused by the guidewire.[23] Because red blood cells attenuate OCT signal, the intensity of signal attenuation can help differentiate red from white thrombi. Red thrombus is composed primarily of red blood cells and therefore appears as a signal-rich mass with high signal attenuation (Fig. 4A). In contrast, white thrombus consists primarily of white blood cells and platelets and therefore appears as a signal-rich mass with low signal attenuation (see Fig. 4B).[24]

Acute Coronary Syndrome

Most acute coronary syndrome presentations are attributable to coronary thrombosis caused by one of three distinct underlying pathologic mechanisms: plaque rupture, plaque erosion, or calcified nodules.[25] In one series of patients presenting with sudden cardiac death, acute coronary thrombosis was attributed to plaque rupture in 60% of cases, plaque erosion in 36% of cases, and calcified nodules in only 4% of cases.[26] The key features of the pathologic definitions of plaque rupture, plaque erosion, and calcified nodule have been used to develop OCT criteria for their diagnosis in vivo (Fig. 5).[27]

Plaque rupture is identified on pathology as an area of fibrous cap disruption with an overlying thrombus that is in continuity with the underlying necrotic core.[26] However, on OCT imaging, overlying thrombus may or may not be seen, because it may have dissolved or embolized distally before OCT imaging. OCT-defined plaque rupture is therefore identified as a lipid plaque with fibrous cap discontinuity and cavity formation inside the plaque (Fig. 6A).[28]

Plaque erosion is challenging to diagnose by OCT. On pathologic analysis, erosion is identified when coronary thrombosis occurs in the absence of fibrous cap disruption; the endothelium lining is commonly absent, and the exposed intima is primarily composed of smooth muscle cells and

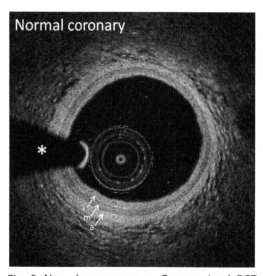

Fig. 2. Normal coronary artery. Cross-sectional OCT image showing the 3-layered structure of a normal coronary arterial wall. a, adventitia; i, intima; m, media. The asterisk denote guidewire shadow artifact.

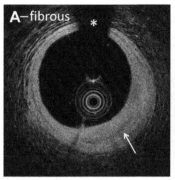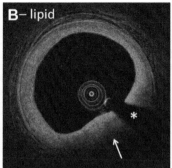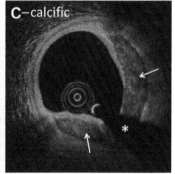

Fig. 3. Plaque characterization. (*A*) Fibrous tissue appears as a homogeneous area of high reflectivity with low signal attenuation (*arrow*). (*B*) Lipid appears as a homogeneous area of low reflectivity with high signal attenuation (*arrow*). (*C*) Calcium appears as a heterogeneous area of high or low reflectivity with low signal attenuation and a sharp demarcating border (*arrows*). The asterisks denote guidewire shadow artifact.

proteoglycan with a paucity of inflammatory cells.[26] OCT imaging is unable to resolve the coronary endothelial lining; thus, alternate criteria have been developed to identify definite and probable OCT-defined erosion. Definite OCT erosion requires the presence of attached thrombus overlying an intact and visualized plaque (see **Fig. 6B**). Probable OCT erosion is defined in the absence of attached thrombus by luminal surface irregularity at the culprit site or in the presence of attached thrombus without underlying plaque by a lack of superficial lipid or calcification in sites adjacent to the culprit lesion.[27]

Calcified nodules are described on pathologic studies as fibrous cap disruption and thrombus overlying a fractured calcified plate.[25,26] On OCT imaging, thrombus may or may not be seen, as is the case with plaque rupture. The OCT definition of calcified nodules describes sites of fibrous cap disruption with underlying calcified plaque characterized by protruding calcification,

superficial calcium, or the presence of significant calcium adjacent to the lesion (see **Fig. 6C**).[27]

Optical Coherence Tomography Features Associated with Vulnerability for Plaque Rupture

The term vulnerable plaque has been used imprecisely to describe plaques that are prone to thrombosis and acute coronary syndrome as well as plaques that are specifically prone to rupture.[25] Although the precursor lesions for luminal thrombosis caused by plaque erosion and calcified nodules should be included as vulnerable plaques, the features that contribute to plaque vulnerability for rupture are the most studied and therefore best understood. The high resolution of OCT imaging makes it a powerful tool in studying and identifying features associated with vulnerability for plaque rupture,[29] including thin fibrous caps, large lipid cores, microchannels, macrophage infiltration,

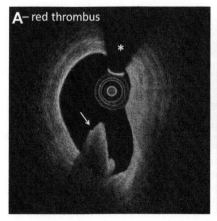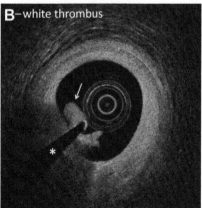

Fig. 4. Thrombus. (*A*) Red thrombus composed primarily of red blood cells appears as a signal-rich mass with high signal attenuation (*arrow*). (*B*) White thrombus composed primarily of white blood cells and platelets appears as a signal-rich mass with low signal attenuation (*arrow*). The asterisks denote guidewire shadow artifact.

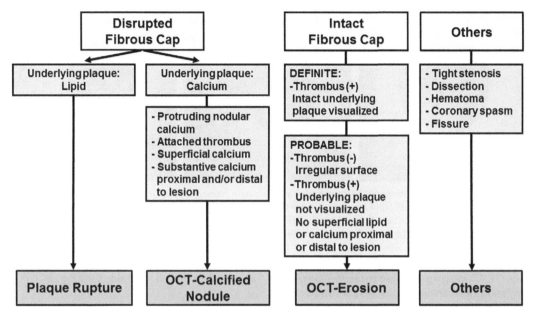

Fig. 5. Algorithm for acute coronary syndrome lesion classification by OCT. (*From* Jia H, Abtahian F, Aguirre AD, et al. In vivo diagnosis of plaque erosion and calcified nodule in patients with acute coronary syndrome by intravascular optical coherence tomography. J Am Coll Cardiol 2013;62(19):1750; with permission.)

superficial spotty calcification, and cholesterol crystals.

Thin-cap fibroatheroma

Thin-cap fibroatheromas (TCFAs) appear morphologically similar to ruptured plaques on pathologic examination and have been postulated to be the precursor lesions for plaque rupture.[25] TCFA are defined as lipid-rich plaque with an overlying fibrous cap measuring less than 65 μm (Fig. 7A). This threshold was derived from a study in which histologic examination of ruptured coronary plaques revealed that 95% had fibrous caps measuring less than 65 μm.[30] On OCT imaging, fibrous tissue appears as a signal-rich area with low signal attenuation, and lipid pools appear as homogeneous signal-poor areas. This sharp contrast in signal intensity between a fibrous cap and underlying lipid makes OCT particularly useful in accurately measuring fibrous cap thickness[31] and thereby identifying TCFA in vivo. One of the first OCT studies comparing plaque characteristics

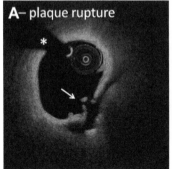
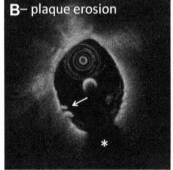
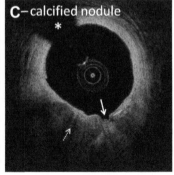

Fig. 6. Acute coronary syndrome. (A) Plaque rupture is defined as a lipid plaque with fibrous cap discontinuity (*arrow*) and cavity formation inside the plaque. (B) Definite plaque erosion is defined by the presence of attached thrombus (*arrow*) overlying an intact and visualized plaque. Probable plaque erosion is identified in the absence of attached thrombus by luminal surface irregularity at the culprit site or in the presence of attached thrombus without underlying plaque by a lack of superficial lipid or calcification in sites adjacent to the culprit lesion. (C) Calcified nodules are defined by fibrous cap disruption (*solid arrow*) with underlying calcified plaque (*dotted arrow*) characterized by protruding calcification, superficial calcium, or the presence of significant calcium adjacent to the lesion. The asterisks denote guidewire shadow artifact.

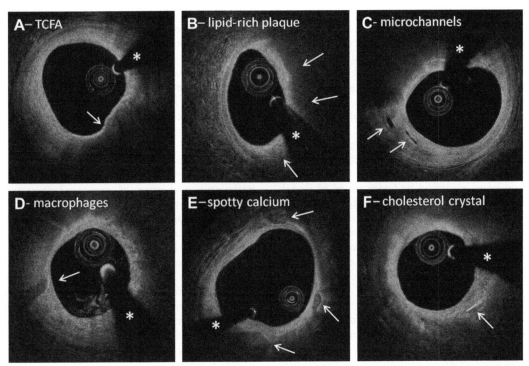

Fig. 7. Features associated with vulnerability for plaque rupture. (*A*) Thin-cap fibroatheroma (TCFA) are defined as lipid-rich plaque with an overlying fibrous cap measuring less than 65 μm (*arrow*). (*B*) Lipid-rich plaque (*arrows*) is defined by lipid occupying 2 or more quadrants of the cross-sectional image. (*C*) Microchannels (*arrows*) are identified as small black (signal absent) holes within a plaque that measure 50 to 300 μm in diameter and span at least 3 consecutive frames on pullback imaging. (*D*) Macrophage accumulations (*arrow*) have been identified as linear series of signal-rich spots with high signal attenuation. (*E*) Spotty calcium describes calcium deposits (*arrows*) with an arc less than 90° (occupying only 1 quadrant of the cross-sectional image). (*F*) Cholesterol crystals have been described as thin, linear, signal-rich structures with low signal attenuation (*arrow*). The asterisks denote guidewire shadow artifact.

in patients with different clinical presentations showed that patients presenting with acute coronary syndrome have thinner fibrous caps and more prevalent TCFA than patients presenting with stable angina.[23]

Extracellular lipid pools

Large extracellular lipid pools are associated with plaque vulnerability for both rupture and thrombosis.[32] Plaque burden, assessed by IVUS imaging, was shown in the PROSPECT (Providing Regional Observations to Study Predictors of Events in the Coronary Tree) study to be an important predictor of an initially nonculprit lesion causing a future cardiovascular event.[33] On OCT imaging, lipid-rich plaques are defined as lipid occupying greater than or equal to 2 quadrants of the cross-sectional image (see Fig. 7B). OCT-identified lipid-rich plaques have been shown to be more prevalent in patients presenting with acute coronary syndrome compared with patients with stable angina.[23] Moreover, in a study of patients presenting with acute coronary syndrome who underwent

3-vessel imaging with OCT and IVUS, ruptured culprit plaques had a greater plaque burden than both ruptured nonculprit plaques and nonruptured TCFA.[34]

Microchannels

Microchannels have been defined as small black (signal absent) holes within a plaque that measure 50 to 300 μm in diameter and span at least 3 consecutive frames on pullback OCT imaging (see Fig. 7C).[13,35] Studies have shown that the presence of microchannels in culprit lesions is associated with a higher incidence of other features associated with plaque vulnerability, such as TCFA and large lipid pools.[35,36] In nonculprit lesions, the presence of microchannels is associated with subsequent plaque progression.[37] In addition, the presence of microchannels in nonculprit lesions may portend a resistance to statin therapy, because plaques with microchannels achieved less fibrous cap thickening in response to statin therapy compared with plaques without microchannels, despite comparable reductions in serum cholesterol levels.[38]

Macrophages

Macrophages have been found to be more prevalent on histologic evaluation of coronary specimens obtained from directional atherectomy procedures in patients with acute coronary syndrome compared with patients with stable angina.[39] In addition, lipid-laden macrophages have also been shown to constitutively produce extracellular matrix-degrading enzymes.[40] Macrophage content may therefore serve as a marker of, and contribute directly to, plaque vulnerability. On OCT imaging, macrophages have been identified as linear series of signal-rich spots with high signal attenuation (see Fig. 7D). Although in practice the identification of macrophages remains challenging, it is possible by detailed examination of OCT images to accurately differentiate fibrous caps with high versus low macrophage content.[14]

Spotty calcium

The role of calcium in plaque vulnerability remains under investigation. Coronary artery calcium scores have been shown to correlate with total atherosclerotic burden but are poorly predictive for acute coronary syndrome. In contrast, IVUS studies focusing on small calcium deposits with an arc less than 90°, termed spotty calcium, suggest that they may serve as a marker for accelerated plaque progression[41] and risk of rupture.[42,43] The size and pattern of vascular calcification may therefore be more predictive of plaque vulnerability than the total burden of calcification. Although calcium is easily identified on IVUS imaging,[44] detailed measurement and characterization of calcium deposits is challenging. The high attenuation of ultrasound signal by calcium limits the visualization of deeper structures and prevents the accurate measurement of calcium depth.[6] In addition, saturation effect from echodense calcifications can make it difficult to evaluate neighboring structures, limiting overall IVUS image analysis.[21] As noted earlier, calcium appears on OCT imaging as a sharply bordered heterogeneous area of either high or low reflectivity with low signal attenuation,[6,20] and deposits occupying only 1 quadrant of the cross-sectional OCT image are identified as spotty calcium (see Fig. 7E). These features make OCT a powerful tool in further characterizing vascular calcifications. For example, the depth of calcium deposits, defined as the minimum distance between the inner edge of the calcium deposit and the luminal surface, can be measured by OCT and may influence plaque vulnerability.[45] TCFA are readily identified by OCT, and

colocalization of spotty calcium deposits and TCFA has been shown to predict procedure-related myocardial injury following elective stent implantation.[46] It is hoped that the high resolution of OCT and lack of significant signal attenuation or saturation artifact on OCT evaluation of calcium will facilitate improved understanding of the role of calcium in plaque progression and vulnerability.

Cholesterol crystals

Cholesterol crystals have been observed on pathologic evaluation of coronary plaques,[26] and crystal content has been shown to correlate with plaque size, plaque disruption, and graded risk of thrombus.[47] On OCT imaging, cholesterol crystals have been described as thin, linear, signal-rich structures with low signal attenuation (see Fig. 7F).[15,48] The presence of cholesterol crystals detected by OCT in the culprit lesions of patients with stable coronary disease has been shown to correlate with the presence of more validated features of plaque vulnerability, such as spotty calcification, microchannels, and lipid-rich plaque.[15]

OPTICAL COHERENCE TOMOGRAPHY IMAGE INTERPRETATION: QUANTITATIVE ANALYSIS

Definitions and methodologies for OCT image–based measurements have been proposed[7,18] and are largely based on the expert consensus document for IVUS-based measurements.[49] The lumen boundary at lesion sites can be traced to derive cross-sectional area, minimum and maximum diameters, and lumen eccentricity. These values can be compared with similar measurements at reference sites, defined both proximally and distally as the site with the largest lumen within 10 mm of the same coronary segment without any major intervening branches, to derive lumen area stenosis.

Note that the deep boundary of plaque is defined differently by OCT compared with IVUS. With IVUS imaging, the internal elastic lamina can be difficult to identify, and the deep boundary of plaque is therefore defined using the external elastic membrane. IVUS-based measurements therefore often include plaque plus media. With OCT imaging, the presence of plaque often obscures the 3-layer structure seen in normal coronary arteries, making plaque burden difficult, if not impossible, to measure. However, when the internal elastic lamina can be seen, OCT-derived plaque measurement corresponds with true histologically defined plaque, as it excludes the muscular media.

Given the limitations of OCT in quantifying plaque burden or demarcating the boundaries of lipid pools, lipid is often quantified by the arc of involvement on circumferential OCT images and by the length of involvement longitudinally. The extent of calcification can be described similarly, although the sharp-bordered appearance of calcium on OCT images enables more detailed measurements to be made as well. Lipid and calcium arc are also often semiquantified as encompassing 1, 2, 3, or 4 quadrants on cross-sectional imaging. The OCT-based definitions of lipid-rich plaque and spotty calcifications use this method of semiquantification.

Stent evaluation is fully reviewed in a separate article in this issue, but OCT may be useful in guiding decision making during coronary intervention.[50] In particular, OCT can be used in the post–percutaneous coronary intervention period for assessment of stent underexpansion, malapposition, tissue protrusion, and edge dissection,[51] and in late stent follow-up for the evaluation of stent strut coverage, degree of neointimal hyperplasia, malapposition, and neoatherosclerosis.[52–54]

ARTIFACTS

An important component of OCT image analysis is the recognition of OCT artifacts that may either mimic or limit identification of true tissue structures (Fig. 8).[11,18]

Artifacts Related to Imaging Technique
Obliquity artifact
Obliquity artifact occurs when the imaging catheter is not parallel to the longitudinal axis of the vessel wall, creating an elliptically distorted off-axis image; this artifact can occur because of vessel curvature or tortuosity and can make measurements less accurate.

Residual blood
Residual blood caused by suboptimal flushing appears as a signal-rich swirling pattern within the lumen and can sometimes be falsely identified as red thrombus. Because red blood cells cause high OCT signal attenuation, residual blood in the vessel lumen may also limit characterization of the underlying tissue.

Artifacts Related to Image Processing
Sew-up artifact
Sew-up artifact (motion artifact) appears as a single radius of misalignment in the circumferential image and results from the rapid movement of the artery or imaging wire.

Nonuniform rotation distortion
Nonuniform rotation distortion appears as smearing within an arc of the circumferential OCT image; it most commonly occurs in the setting of vessel tortuosity, tight stenosis, heavy calcification, or equipment imperfections that perturb the smooth rotation of the optical components, resulting in variation in the rotational speed of the imaging catheter.

Fold-over artifact
Fold-over artifact occurs with FD-OCT imaging systems when reflected signals from structures beyond the system's field of view produce aliasing along the Fourier transformation, causing a portion of the vessel to appear to fold over in the image; this artifact occurs most commonly at side branches or with large vessels.

Artifacts Related to the Imaging Catheter or Guidewire
Shadow artifact
Shadow artifact appears as a reduction in signal intensity beyond a structure such as a guidewire or metallic stent strut, or small bubbles in the imaging catheter. As detailed earlier, blood, thrombus, and macrophage accumulations can also attenuate the OCT signal, limiting the evaluation of underlying structures.

Multiple reflections
Multiple reflections appear as 1 or more circles centered on the imaging catheter and result from reflections from multiple facets of the catheter.

Artifacts Related to Stent Struts
Reverberation artifact
Reverberation artifact is similar to the multiple reflections artifact and describes reflections produced by stent struts that are centered on the imaging catheter.

Saturation artifact
Saturation artifact occurs when stent struts or other highly reflective structures produce a high-amplitude backscattered signal that is beyond the range that can be accurately detected by the data acquisition system; this artifact appears as spokes of high and low intensity signal emanating from the center of the imaging catheter and passing through the highly reflective structure.

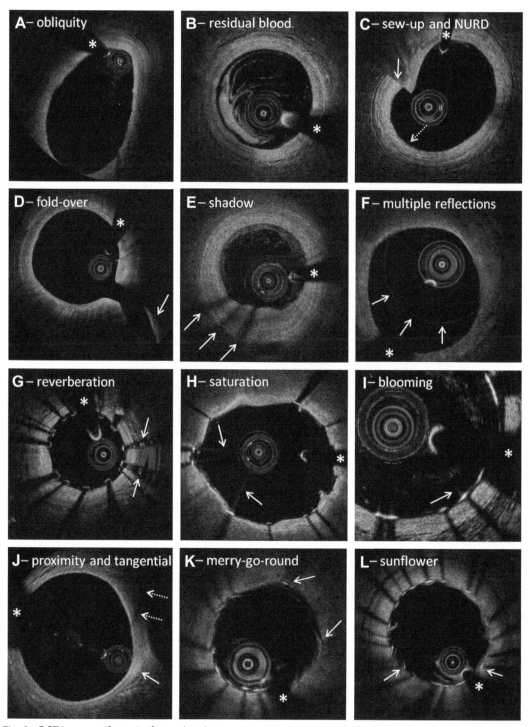

Fig. 8. OCT image artifacts. Artifacts related to imaging technique include obliquity artifact (*A*) and residual blood (*B*). Artifacts related to image processing include sew-up artifact (*C, solid arrow*), nonuniform rotation distortion (*C, dotted arrow*), and fold-over artifact (*arrow in D*). Artifacts related to the imaging catheter or guidewire include shadowing (*arrows in E*) and multiple reflections (*arrows in F*). Artifacts related to stent struts include reverberation (*arrows in G*), saturation (*arrows in H*), and blooming (*arrows in I*). Artifacts related to eccentric wire position include proximity artifact (*J, solid arrow*), tangential signal dropout (*J, dotted arrows*), merry-go-round effect (*arrows in K*), and sunflower effect (*arrows in L*). The asterisks denote guidewire shadow artifact.

Blooming artifact
Blooming artifact occurs when stent struts or other highly reflective structures appear slightly smeared or thickened in the axial direction.

Artifacts Related to Eccentric Wire Position
Proximity artifact
Proximity artifact can occur when the imaging catheter is near or touching the artery wall, causing the adjacent tissue to appear brighter or more signal rich.

Tangential signal dropout
Tangential signal dropout also occurs when the imaging catheter is near or touching the artery wall and appears as attenuated signal tangential to the luminal surface.

Merry-go-round effect
Merry-go-round effect is a term used to describe the reduced lateral resolution at increased distances or depths from the imaging catheter. Stent struts offer the most easily recognized example of the merry-go-round effect, because struts that are farther from the imaging catheter encompass a wider arc, appearing wider than struts closer to the imaging catheter.

Sunflower effect
Sunflower effect (also called strut orientation artifact) describes the artificial alignment of reflections from stent struts toward the imaging catheter, mimicking the way sunflowers align toward the sun. At its extreme, this type of artifact can cause stent struts to appear almost perpendicular to the lumen surface in order to align towards the eccentrically positioned catheter.

SUMMARY

Intravascular imaging with OCT has proved to be a robust tool for studying the mechanisms underlying plaque formation and acute coronary syndrome. The high resolution of OCT imaging derives from its use of light waves rather than ultrasound waves, and enables real-time tissue characterization in vivo. Although the limited depth of penetration of OCT imaging may limit the assessment of plaque burden and deep tissue structures, prior work has validated the ability of OCT to accurately discriminate different types of plaque and to identify features associated with plaque vulnerability for thrombosis and rupture, which are predominantly located in the superficial part of the vessel. Studies are now underway investigating the use of OCT in guiding clinical decision making,[55] and further improvements in OCT technology should expand its utility in both research and clinical settings.

REFERENCES

1. Huang D, Swanson EA, Lin CP, et al. Optical coherence tomography. Science 1991;254(5035): 1178–81.
2. Adhi M, Duker JS. Optical coherence tomography–current and future applications. Curr Opin Ophthalmol 2013;24(3):213–21.
3. Brezinski ME, Tearney GJ, Bouma BE, et al. Optical coherence tomography for optical biopsy. Properties and demonstration of vascular pathology. Circulation 1996;93(6):1206–13.
4. Abtahian F, Jang IK. Optical coherence tomography: basics, current application and future potential. Curr Opin Pharmacol 2012;12(5):583–91.
5. Bouma BE, Yun SH, Vakoc BJ, et al. Fourier-domain optical coherence tomography: recent advances toward clinical utility. Curr Opin Biotechnol 2009; 20(1):111–8.
6. Jang IK, Bouma BE, Kang DH, et al. Visualization of coronary atherosclerotic plaques in patients using optical coherence tomography: comparison with intravascular ultrasound. J Am Coll Cardiol 2002; 39(4):604–9.
7. Prati F, Regar E, Mintz GS, et al. Expert review document on methodology, terminology, and clinical applications of optical coherence tomography: physical principles, methodology of image acquisition, and clinical application for assessment of coronary arteries and atherosclerosis. Eur Heart J 2010;31(4):401–15.
8. Yamaguchi T, Terashima M, Akasaka T, et al. Safety and feasibility of an intravascular optical coherence tomography image wire system in the clinical setting. Am J Cardiol 2008;101(5):562–7.
9. Kim SJ, Lee H, Kato K, et al. In vivo comparison of lumen dimensions measured by time domain-, and frequency domain-optical coherence tomography, and intravascular ultrasound. Int J Cardiovasc Imaging 2013;29(5):967–75.
10. Prati F, Cera M, Ramazzotti V, et al. Safety and feasibility of a new non-occlusive technique for facilitated intracoronary optical coherence tomography (OCT) acquisition in various clinical and anatomical scenarios. EuroIntervention 2007;3(3): 365–70.
11. Bezerra HG, Costa MA, Guagliumi G, et al. Intracoronary optical coherence tomography: a comprehensive review clinical and research applications. JACC Cardiovasc Interv 2009;2(11):1035–46.
12. Suh WM, Seto AH, Margey RJ, et al. Intravascular detection of the vulnerable plaque. Circ Cardiovasc Imaging 2011;4(2):169–78.

13. Vorpahl M, Nakano M, Virmani R. Small black holes in optical frequency domain imaging matches intravascular neoangiogenesis formation in histology. Eur Heart J 2010;31(15):1889.

14. Tearney GJ, Yabushita H, Houser SL, et al. Quantification of macrophage content in atherosclerotic plaques by optical coherence tomography. Circulation 2003;107(1):113–9.

15. Nakamura S, Inami S, Murai K, et al. Relationship between cholesterol crystals and culprit lesion characteristics in patients with stable coronary artery disease: an optical coherence tomography study. Clin Res Cardiol 2014;103:1015–21.

16. Lowe HC, Narula J, Fujimoto JG, et al. Intracoronary optical diagnostics current status, limitations, and potential. JACC Cardiovasc Interv 2011;4(12):1257–70.

17. Prati F, Guagliumi G, Mintz GS, et al. Expert review document part 2: methodology, terminology and clinical applications of optical coherence tomography for the assessment of interventional procedures. Eur Heart J 2012;33(20):2513–20.

18. Tearney GJ, Regar E, Akasaka T, et al. Consensus standards for acquisition, measurement, and reporting of intravascular optical coherence tomography studies: a report from the International Working Group for Intravascular Optical Coherence Tomography Standardization and Validation. J Am Coll Cardiol 2012;59(12):1058–72.

19. Di Vito L, Yoon JH, Kato K, et al. Comprehensive overview of definitions for optical coherence tomography-based plaque and stent analyses. Coron Artery Dis 2014;25(2):172–85.

20. Yabushita H, Bouma BE, Houser SL, et al. Characterization of human atherosclerosis by optical coherence tomography. Circulation 2002;106(13):1640–5.

21. Kume T, Akasaka T, Kawamoto T, et al. Assessment of coronary arterial plaque by optical coherence tomography. Am J Cardiol 2006;97(8):1172–5.

22. Manfrini O, Mont E, Leone O, et al. Sources of error and interpretation of plaque morphology by optical coherence tomography. Am J Cardiol 2006; 98(2):156–9.

23. Jang IK, Tearney GJ, MacNeill B, et al. In vivo characterization of coronary atherosclerotic plaque by use of optical coherence tomography. Circulation 2005;111(12):1551–5.

24. Kume T, Akasaka T, Kawamoto T, et al. Assessment of coronary arterial thrombus by optical coherence tomography. Am J Cardiol 2006;97(12):1713–7.

25. Virmani R, Burke AP, Farb A, et al. Pathology of the vulnerable plaque. J Am Coll Cardiol 2006; 47(Suppl 8):C13–8.

26. Virmani R, Kolodgie FD, Burke AP, et al. Lessons from sudden coronary death: a comprehensive morphological classification scheme for atherosclerotic lesions. Arterioscler Thromb Vasc Biol 2000; 20(5):1262–75.

27. Jia H, Abtahian F, Aguirre AD, et al. In vivo diagnosis of plaque erosion and calcified nodule in patients with acute coronary syndrome by intravascular optical coherence tomography. J Am Coll Cardiol 2013;62(19):1748–58.

28. Kubo T, Imanishi T, Takarada S, et al. Assessment of culprit lesion morphology in acute myocardial infarction: ability of optical coherence tomography compared with intravascular ultrasound and coronary angioscopy. J Am Coll Cardiol 2007;50(10): 933–9.

29. Kato K, Yasutake M, Yonetsu T, et al. Intracoronary imaging modalities for vulnerable plaques. J Nippon Med Sch 2011;78(6):340–51.

30. Burke AP, Farb A, Malcolm GT, et al. Coronary risk factors and plaque morphology in men with coronary disease who died suddenly. N Engl J Med 1997;336(18):1276–82.

31. Kume T, Akasaka T, Kawamoto T, et al. Measurement of the thickness of the fibrous cap by optical coherence tomography. Am Heart J 2006;152(4): 755.e1–4.

32. Davies MJ, Richardson PD, Woolf N, et al. Risk of thrombosis in human atherosclerotic plaques: role of extracellular lipid, macrophage, and smooth muscle cell content. Br Heart J 1993;69(5):377–81.

33. Stone GW, Maehara A, Lansky AJ, et al. A prospective natural-history study of coronary atherosclerosis. N Engl J Med 2011;364(3):226–35.

34. Tian J, Ren X, Vergallo R, et al. Distinct morphological features of ruptured culprit plaque for acute coronary events compared to those with silent rupture and thin-cap fibroatheroma: a combined optical coherence tomography and intravascular ultrasound study. J Am Coll Cardiol 2014;63(21):2209–16.

35. Kitabata H, Tanaka A, Kubo T, et al. Relation of microchannel structure identified by optical coherence tomography to plaque vulnerability in patients with coronary artery disease. Am J Cardiol 2010;105(12):1673–8.

36. Tian J, Hou J, Xing L, et al. Significance of intraplaque neovascularisation for vulnerability: optical coherence tomography study. Heart 2012;98(20): 1504–9.

37. Uemura S, Ishigami K, Soeda T, et al. Thin-cap fibroatheroma and microchannel findings in optical coherence tomography correlate with subsequent progression of coronary atheromatous plaques. Eur Heart J 2012;33(1):78–85.

38. Tian J, Hou J, Xing L, et al. Does neovascularization predict response to statin therapy? Optical coherence tomography study. Int J Cardiol 2012;158: 469–70.

39. Moreno PR, Falk E, Palacios IF, et al. Macrophage infiltration in acute coronary syndromes. Implications for plaque rupture. Circulation 1994;90(2): 775–8.

40. Galis ZS, Sukhova GK, Kranzhofer R, et al. Macrophage foam cells from experimental atheroma constitutively produce matrix-degrading proteinases. Proc Natl Acad Sci U S A 1995;92(2):402–6.

41. Kataoka Y, Wolski K, Uno K, et al. Spotty calcification as a marker of accelerated progression of coronary atherosclerosis: insights from serial intravascular ultrasound. J Am Coll Cardiol 2012; 59(18):1592–7.

42. Ehara S, Kobayashi Y, Yoshiyama M, et al. Spotty calcification typifies the culprit plaque in patients with acute myocardial infarction: an intravascular ultrasound study. Circulation 2004;110(22):3424–9.

43. Fujii K, Carlier SG, Mintz GS, et al. Intravascular ultrasound study of patterns of calcium in ruptured coronary plaques. Am J Cardiol 2005;96(3):352–7.

44. Mintz GS, Douek P, Pichard AD, et al. Target lesion calcification in coronary artery disease: an intravascular ultrasound study. J Am Coll Cardiol 1992; 20(5):1149–55.

45. Mizukoshi M, Kubo T, Takarada S, et al. Coronary superficial and spotty calcium deposits in culprit coronary lesions of acute coronary syndrome as determined by optical coherence tomography. Am J Cardiol 2013;112(1):34–40.

46. Ueda T, Uemura S, Watanabe M, et al. Colocalization of thin-cap fibroatheroma and spotty calcification is a powerful predictor of procedure-related myocardial injury after elective coronary stent implantation. Coron Artery Dis 2014;25(5):384–91.

47. Abela GS, Aziz K, Vedre A, et al. Effect of cholesterol crystals on plaques and intima in arteries of patients with acute coronary and cerebrovascular syndromes. Am J Cardiol 2009;103(7):959–68.

48. Liu L, Gardecki JA, Nadkarni SK, et al. Imaging the subcellular structure of human coronary atherosclerosis using micro-optical coherence tomography. Nat Med 2011;17(8):1010–4.

49. Mintz GS, Nissen SE, Anderson WD, et al. American College of Cardiology Clinical Expert Consensus Document on Standards for Acquisition, Measurement and Reporting of Intravascular Ultrasound Studies (IVUS). A report of the American College of Cardiology Task Force on Clinical Expert Consensus Documents. J Am Coll Cardiol 2001;37(5):1478–92.

50. Prati F, Di Vito L, Biondi-Zoccai G, et al. Angiography alone versus angiography plus optical coherence tomography to guide decision-making during percutaneous coronary intervention: the Centro per la Lotta contro l'Infarto-Optimisation of Percutaneous Coronary Intervention (CLI-OPCI) study. EuroIntervention 2012;8(7):823–9.

51. Bouma BE, Tearney GJ, Yabushita H, et al. Evaluation of intracoronary stenting by intravascular optical coherence tomography. Heart 2003;89(3): 317–20.

52. Gonzalo N, Serruys PW, Okamura T, et al. Optical coherence tomography patterns of stent restenosis. Am Heart J 2009;158(2):284–93.

53. Takano M, Yamamoto M, Inami S, et al. Appearance of lipid-laden intima and neovascularization after implantation of bare-metal stents extended late-phase observation by intracoronary optical coherence tomography. J Am Coll Cardiol 2009; 55(1):26–32.

54. Kang SJ, Mintz GS, Akasaka T, et al. Optical coherence tomographic analysis of in-stent neoatherosclerosis after drug-eluting stent implantation. Circulation 2011;123(25):2954–63.

55. Souteyrand G, Amabile N, Combaret N, et al. Invasive management without stents in selected acute coronary syndrome patients with a large thrombus burden: a prospective study of optical coherence tomography guided treatment decisions. EuroIntervention 2014. [Epub ahead of print].

Technical Considerations and Practical Guidance for Intracoronary Optical Coherence Tomography

CrossMark

Arabindra B. Katwal, MBBS, John J. Lopez, MD*

KEYWORDS

- Intravascular imaging • Optical coherence tomography • Coronary intervention

KEY POINTS

- Optical coherence tomography (OCT) is an intravascular imaging technology analogous to intravascular ultrasound (IVUS), using near-infrared light rather than ultrasound, thereby providing higher-resolution images.
- Successful OCT image acquisition requires adequate positioning of the imaging catheter and sufficient luminal blood clearance with contrast injection.
- Guide catheter size should generally be at least 6F, and the guide catheter shape should provide well-seated, coaxial alignment with the coronary ostium.
- For power injection, specific settings for the left and right coronary arteries should be used.
- Relevant OCT measurements before percutaneous coronary intervention (PCI) include lesion length, minimal luminal area, proximal and distal reference vessel locations, and diameters.
- Relevant post-PCI OCT assessment includes stent expansion, apposition, edge dissection, plaque prolapse, and geographic miss.
- Successful, safe, and efficient OCT imaging requires an understanding of the system setup, imaging catheter characteristics, and methods to improve image quality.

INTRODUCTION

OCT is a recently established modality for intracoronary imaging. Although initially developed for in vivo retinal imaging, OCT has, after nearly 2 decades of research, evolved into a clinically applicable diagnostic tool for interventional cardiology. OCT uses light in the near-infrared spectrum (wavelength 1250–1350 nm) to provide a large amount of qualitative and quantitative information regarding vessel lumen diameter, plaque morphology, lesion length, and lesion characteristics. In so doing, it is an important tool to guide PCI strategy. The wavelength range used by OCT permits adequate tissue penetration with an axial resolution of 12 to 18 µm and a lateral resolution of 20 to 90 µm (as a function of distance from the arterial wall). This degree of resolution is approximately 10-fold higher than that of IVUS.[1] This review provides a practical guide to OCT imaging, with a particular emphasis on the techniques and approaches to optimize image acquisition, improve the evaluation of coronary lesions, and guide the strategies for PCI.

The authors have nothing to disclose.
Division of Cardiology, Department of Medicine, Stritch School of Medicine, Loyola University Medical Center, 2160 South First Avenue, Maywood, IL 60153, USA
* Corresponding author. Loyola University Medical Center, 2160 South First Avenue, Building No. 110, Room No. 6289, Maywood, IL 60153.
E-mail address: jlopez7@LUMC.edu

Intervent Cardiol Clin 4 (2015) 239–249
http://dx.doi.org/10.1016/j.iccl.2015.02.005
2211-7458/15/$ – see front matter © 2015 Elsevier Inc. All rights reserved.

OPTICAL COHERENCE TOMOGRAPHY SYSTEMS AVAILABLE IN THE UNITED STATES AT PRESENT

Coronary OCT systems in their first incarnation were time-domain (TD) systems that required balloon occlusion to provide the blood-free lumen necessary to acquire adequate images. These systems are now of only historical interest, because they have been supplanted by the development of frequency/Fourier-domain (FD) systems, which can rapidly acquire images and therefore enable the use of contrast injection to clear luminal blood, eliminating the need for balloon occlusion. The ILUMIEN and ILUMIEN OPTIS systems (St. Jude Medical, Inc, Westford MA, USA) are OCT-FD systems that are approved for use by the US Food and Drug Administration (FDA). These systems rapidly image along a relatively long segment of vessel in 3 seconds or less. The OPTIS system has 2 modes of image acquisition: survey and high resolution. The survey mode provides a rapid pullback of 75 mm over 2.1 seconds at 180 frames per second (ie, in 5 frames/mm). The high-resolution mode images a 54-mm vessel segment at a similar frame rate over 3 seconds (ie, 10 frames/mm), which provides twice the frame density with the same pullback length and duration as the original ILUMIEN system (Table 1). The OPTIS system software also provides an automated lumen profile that can improve stent planning workflow, such as automatic lumen detection on every frame, a profile of mean diameter or area across the length of the pullback, automatic marking of the site of the minimal lumen area (MLA), and automated display of reference frame areas and diameters.

Table 1
Characteristics of OCT image acquisition with the ILUMIEN OPTIS system

Parameter	Survey Mode	High-Resolution Mode
Engine speed	180 frames/s	180 frames/s
Pullback speed	36 mm/s	18 mm/s
Frame density	5 frames/mm	10 frames/mm
Pullback length	75 mm	54 mm
Pullback duration	2.1 s	3.0 s
Total frames collected	375 frames	540 frames

In addition, the high-resolution mode allows for real-time, immediate 3-dimensional reconstruction of the vessel lumen, which aids in the analysis of complex anatomy.

CLINICAL APPLICATION OF INTRACORONARY OPTICAL COHERENCE TOMOGRAPHY

In 2010, the FDA approved OCT for imaging within native coronary arteries 2.0 mm to 3.5 mm in diameter. The 2011 American College of Cardiology Foundation/American Heart Association/Society of Cardiovascular Angiography and Interventions Guideline for PCI does not provide formal recommendations regarding the clinical use of OCT, in contrast to IVUS.[2] Despite the lack of formal recommendations, OCT is increasingly being used in a variety of clinical scenarios similar to guideline-directed IVUS imaging largely based on recent data, published consensus documents, and extrapolation from the IVUS literature. Key applications for OCT include evaluating nonostial lesions that are angiographically intermediate in severity, guiding coronary stent implantation, and assessing the mechanism of stent thrombosis or restenosis.

Optical Coherence Tomography for the Assessment of Coronary Stenosis Severity

Fractional flow reserve (FFR) has become the gold standard to determine the physiologic significance of coronary stenoses.[3,4] Nonetheless, the measurement of MLA by IVUS is also widely used to further evaluate the severity of angiographically intermediate coronary lesions. The basis for this approach comes from several studies that have shown moderate correlations between IVUS-derived MLA measurements and FFR values, with receiver operator characteristic (ROC) area under the curve (AUC) values ranging between 0.68 and 0.80.[5–7] Furthermore, an IVUS-based approach has been associated with good clinical outcomes and low subsequent adverse event rates.[8] OCT, similar to IVUS, can provide highly accurate and reproducible lumen area measurements.[9] The relationships between OCT-derived MLA, IVUS-derived MLA, and FFR have also been examined.[10] The optimal cutoff to predict an FFR less than or equal to 0.80 was an OCT-derived MLA threshold less than or equal to 1.95 mm^2, which provided a sensitivity of 82%, specificity of 67%, positive predictive value of 68%, and negative predictive value of 80%. Owing to only moderate specificity and a modest positive predictive value, an OCT-derived MLA less than or equal to 1.95 mm^2 cannot solely be used to justify intervention in the absence of additional functional assessment. Lesions with an OCT-derived MLA greater than 1.95 mm^2 are unlikely to be hemodynamically significant, based on the moderate sensitivity (82%) and negative predictive value of this threshold (80%). An MLA threshold of 1.62 mm^2 may be more appropriate in small vessels less than 3.0 mm in diameter; according to ROC curve analysis, this threshold has a significantly higher AUC to predict a significant FFR compared with IVUS (0.77 vs 0.63, $P = .04$).

However, given the presence of robust clinical evidence for physiologic lesion assessment with FFR, the use of OCT-derived anatomic criteria as a surrogate for functional significance should not be a standard approach.[5–7] In addition, the safety and efficacy of a strategy of performing PCI based on OCT-derived MLA less than or equal to 1.95 mm^2 and deferring PCI in the setting of an MLA greater than 1.95 mm^2 has not been determined. Larger and adequately powered studies are needed to define and validate optimal OCT-derived MLA thresholds against FFR.

Optical Coherence Tomography for Guiding Stent Implantation

This topic is discussed in detail elsewhere in this issue by Guagliumi and colleagues. In brief, given the excellent spatial resolution of OCT compared with IVUS, OCT imaging is ideally suited to guide PCI of nonostial lesions. The advantages of OCT in this setting include reproducible and accurate lesion length and reference vessel luminal measurements to guide stent selection, the ability to characterize plaque components to determine the risk of periprocedural myocardial infarction,[11–13] the potential ability to identify and avoid "geographic miss" related to partial coverage of higher-risk lipid plaque locations, and optimizing stent results by identifying stent underexpansion, malapposition, and edge dissection.[14–16]

Optical Coherence Tomography for the Assessment of Stent Thrombosis and Restenosis

This topic is covered in detail elsewhere in this issue by Parodi and colleagues and Hong and colleagues. In brief, the high resolution of OCT to detect malapposition and stent fracture, and to characterize and accurately quantify tissue ingrowth, may provide important information regarding the mechanism of stent failure and can aid in determining a targeted treatment approach.

TECHNICAL APPROACH TO OPTICAL COHERENCE TOMOGRAPHY IMAGING

Catheter Setup

A 6F catheter or a larger guide introduced via either the radial or the femoral approach is generally used, although 5F guiding catheters have been used successfully by some operators. The major limitation of a 5F guide is that it is more difficult to deliver contrast around the OCT catheter, making it challenging to clear blood from the coronary lumen during the pullback of the OCT imaging element. A rapid exchange imaging catheter is advanced over a 0.014-inch guidewire to the desired imaging location.[17] In the case of the FDA-approved 2.7F monorail C7 Dragonfly and Dragonfly Duo intravascular imaging catheters (Fig. 1) (St. Jude Medical, Inc), the device is first flushed (purged) through its proximal side port with full-strength contrast using a 3-mL syringe. This procedure is required to deair the sheath around the imaging core and to reduce the likelihood of blood entry into the sheath. An air- and blood-free imaging environment is critical to prevent shadow and attenuation artifacts, respectively. The proximal end of the sterile disposable

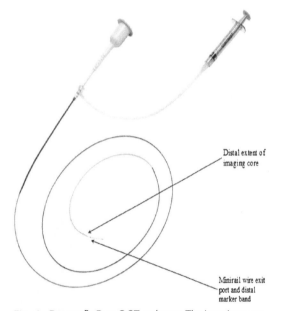

Distal extent of imaging core

Minirail wire exit port and distal marker band

Fig. 1. Dragonfly Duo OCT catheter. The imaging core extends to the distal end 30 mm from the catheter tip, just proximal to the minirail exit port. There are 3 radiopaque markers: the most distal is 4 mm from the catheter tip; the second, a lens marker is just proximal to the imaging element; and the third is 50 mm proximal to the lens marker. (C7 Dragonfly, ILUMIEN, PCI Optimization and St. Jude Medical are trademarks of St. Jude Medical, Inc. or its related companies. Reprinted with permission of St. Jude Medical, © 2014. All rights reserved.)

imaging catheter is then connected to a nonsterile motorized automated docking unit placed with a sterile sheath. The docking unit connects to the wheel-around console that houses the light source, processor, keyboard, and video screen display. The video screen simultaneously displays cross-sectional and longitudinal views of the vessel during imaging (Fig. 2). The system automatically calibrates the catheter once the imaging catheter is connected to the viewing console and flushed. An integrated system is also commercially available that eliminates the wheel-around console and allows the operator to manipulate the acquired images that are displayed on the fluoroscopy boom using a joystick mounted on the side of the patient table. Once the catheter has been connected to the docking unit, the Live View mode is activated by the touch of a button to verify that the catheter components are functioning appropriately. The system is then put on Standby until the catheter is delivered to the targeted location, to prevent catheter damage and to preclude red blood cells from getting trapped within the catheter's housing sheath during advancement through the coronary guide and target vessel.

Catheter Positioning Within the Target Vessel

The distal tip of the C7 Dragonfly catheter has 2 radiopaque markers 20 mm apart representing the catheter tip and the wire exit port. The imaging lens is approximately 5 mm proximal to the wire exit port. Therefore, the wire exit marker must be delivered at least 5 to 7 mm distal to the target site to ensure that the optical lens is past the target lesion. This imaging lens can also be visualized under fluoroscopy. The next-generation Dragonfly Duo catheter has 3 markers (distal tip, imaging lens, and proximal pullback marker located 50 mm proximal to the imaging lens), which permits even easier identification of the imaging lens location and allows the operator to flank the area of interest with the 2 proximal markers, because this demarcates the approximate length of a high-resolution imaging run (see Fig. 1). The lens and 50-mm markers are integrated within the imaging core itself and therefore track with the movement of the imaging lens during pullback.

Image Acquisition

After positioning the imaging catheter to the target location, the Live View mode is activated and the system is autocalibrated. Imaging is initiated by pressing the Enable button on the docking unit or console. The operator then has 15 seconds to create a blood-free lumen by injecting contrast through the guiding catheter, which then triggers automatic catheter pullback.

Preparation for Measurements

Before interpreting the image, the catheter calibration is fine-tuned using the zero-point setting of the system (z-offset) before further interpretation. This off-line manual adjustment is essential for accurate measurements performed on the cross-sectional image along the entire longitudinal imaging segment. This calibration corrects for small variations in optical path lengths by aligning 4 fiduciary marks to match the outer surface of the imaging catheter (Fig. 3). Incorrect

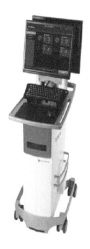
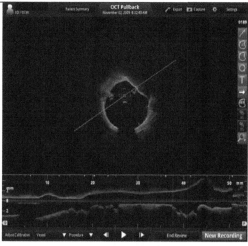

Fig. 2. ILUMIEN Optical Coherence Tomography System and video display screen allowing both cross-sectional (B-mode) and longitudinal (L-mode) vessel views. (C7 Dragonfly, ILUMIEN, PCI Optimization and St. Jude Medical are trademarks of St. Jude Medical, Inc. or its related companies. Reprinted with permission of St. Jude Medical, © 2014. All rights reserved.)

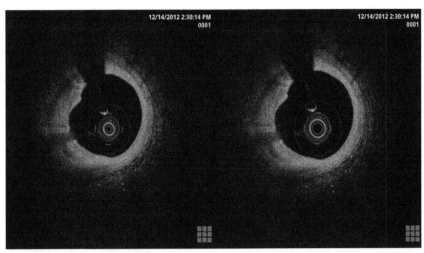

Fig. 3. Incorrect (*left image*) and correct (*right image*) off-line manual calibration of z-point adjustment for catheter size calibration to allow for accurate vessel measurements.

sizing and image misinterpretation may occur without this calibration.[1,18]

Coregistration with Coronary Angiography

The integrated OPTIS system enables the OCT pullback to be coregistered with the coronary angiogram; this allows the operator to clearly understand where the position of a specific frame of the OCT run sits along the angiogram of the vessel. The workflow differs slightly from that of the mobile, nonintegrated unit. The OCT catheter is advanced over the coronary guidewire so that the lens marker is distal to the area of interest. A fluoroscopic projection is chosen that minimizes vessel foreshortening and overlap with other branches. The Live View button on the docking unit is pressed, and adequate blood clearance is confirmed with a puff of contrast through the guide catheter. The Enable button on the docking unit is then pressed, which autocalibrates the catheter; Enable is pressed once more, and the system is ready for image acquisition. The cineangiography pedal of the fluoroscopy system is pressed and held, and then the operator or technician injects contrast to clear the lumen, triggering automatic pullback. The cineangiography pedal is released after the pullback is complete. Using the tabletop joystick controller, the operator or technician marks the distal and proximal points of the target vessel. The software then identifies the target vessel and coregisters the OCT data set with the angiogram. Manipulation of the cursor along the length of the OCT longitudinal view with the tabletop controller now moves a white hash mark along the corresponding position of the angiogram (Fig. 4).

TIPS FOR OPTIMAL IMAGE ACQUISITION

Guiding Catheter Considerations

Optimal guide catheter selection is crucial for procedural success by ensuring the creation of the blood-free field. Swirling due to the presence of red blood cells in the imaging field can compromise image quality, resulting in an inability to interpret the findings or mistaking luminal blood artifact for thrombus (Fig. 5). An optimally shaped and positioned guide catheter will be coaxial with the coronary ostium and deeply engaged without causing ventricularization and/or dampening of pressure waveform.[19] Activating the Live View mode and demonstrating efficient blood clearance from the lumen by manually injecting a small bolus of contrast can be used to confirm correct guide catheter position.[20] This small puff of contrast also purges the guide and manifold tubing of any blood so that no blood is mixed in with the contrast injection. Finally, intracoronary nitroglycerin is recommended before imaging to prevent catheter-induced vasospasm and to allow for accurate vessel sizing.

While 6F is the standard recommended minimal guide catheter size, 5F guiding catheters have been shown to safely obtain high-quality OCT images. Power injection is recommended with a 5F guide, because manual contrast injection through the guide around the imaging catheter is not often possible. The injection rate and duration described below are usually adequate.

Flushing Options to Create a Blood-Free Lumen

Animal studies have shown that higher-viscosity flush solutions provide superior imaging quality

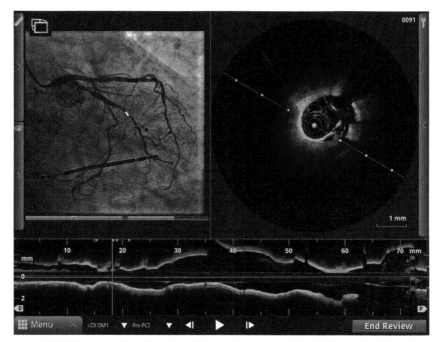

Fig. 4. Integrated OPTIS system. Coregistration of the angiogram and the OCT run identifies the angiographic position of the OCT frame of interest. In this case, a patient presented with a non-ST-elevation acute coronary syndrome, and cardiac catheterization showed a lesion in the first obtuse marginal of indeterminate angiographic severity. OCT on survey mode (75-mm-length pullback) demonstrated rupture of a thin cap fibroatheroma with superimposed nonocclusive platelet-rich thrombus. Lower panel: longitudinal view of OCT. Blue and yellow vertical line demarcates frame of interest. Upper right quadrant: cross-sectional OCT image of frame of interest. Upper left quadrant: angiogram acquired during OCT pullback. White hash mark demarcates frame of interest.

compared with lower-viscosity ones. High-viscosity contrast agents have demonstrated excellent image quality in humans. Iodixanol is the most viscous contrast agent and remains the one of choice.[17–24] Recently, 3 human studies have shown that the quality of image produced by FD-OCT was comparable with that produced using contrast media or low-molecular-weight dextran L (LMD-L).[20,21,23] LMD-L may thus be an acceptable and safe alternative to contrast agents for FD-OCT, although at present only contrast media is approved by the FDA for OCT image acquisition.

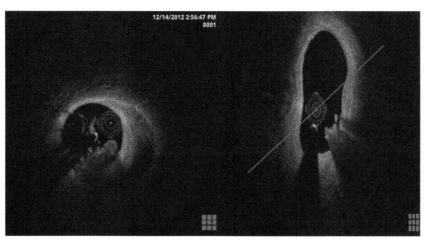

Fig. 5. Creation of blood-free field for imaging is required to avoid blood swirling artifact (*left image*), which can sometimes be confused with luminal thrombus (*right image*).

Most operators in the United States use undiluted contrast material. Despite concerns for reduced viscosity and image quality, there have been reports of adequate image quality with both a 50:50 combination of a crystalloid with contrast during manual injections[22] and power injection of lactated Ringers solution alone without any mixed contrast.[24]

Manual or Power Injection

Both manual and power injection of flushing media resulted in similar blood-free vessel lumen in the early TD-OCT studies.[25–28] In contrast, with current FD-OCT systems, power injections are more reliable in providing a blood-free lumen; this is because of a more consistent rate, duration, and volume of injection.[29] The safety, efficacy, and advantages of power injection for coronary angiography have been previously described.[30,31] Some operators use a manual injection of a combination of saline and contrast because the decreased viscosity results in less difficulty in injection and allows for a good injection rate for an adequate duration to acquire high-quality images.

Optimal Settings for Power Injection

Irrespective of the mode of injection, a low flow rate leads to blood in the viewing field and loss of image quality (Table 2). To avoid this, the recommended power injection settings for current OCT systems are 4 mL/s for the left coronary artery and 3 mL/s for the right coronary artery,[20,32] with a maximum pressure setting of 300 psi, although 400 psi has been used without complications.[23] A nonlinear rise prevents streaming; however, this may dislodge the guide or cause guide catheter recoil during injection, which can lead to blood artifact. If this occurs, a linear rise of 0.3 may help keep the guiding catheter engaged throughout the duration of injection. The injection period should be 4 seconds, with an increase to 5 seconds in the case of any proximal vessel blood artifact at the end of the injection period. When blood clearance is inadequate, a 0.5- to 1.0-mL/s increase in the flow rate can dramatically improve blood clearance.

Large Reference Vessel Diameter

Although the imaging diameter of current OCT catheters is 10.5 mm in saline, the actual upper limit of imaging depth in vivo is 5 to 6 mm because of light absorption and scattering that occurs with tissue penetration. As such, larger vessels are not adequately visualized by OCT, especially if the catheter assumes an eccentric position within the vessel limiting the scan depth on the contralateral vessel wall.

OTHER CONSIDERATIONS

Time

OCT imaging can be routinely performed efficiently, with an average time of less than 4 minutes from setup to completion of image acquisition.[33] This limited incremental time cost should not adversely affect case turnover times for even the busiest of catheterization laboratories. Good coordination between the operator and a well-trained technical staff greatly helps in achieving the goal of efficient OCT imaging.

Safety

The excellent safety profile of FD-OCT using automated power injection technique has been well documented.[23,32–34] Reported adverse events are uncommon and include transient chest discomfort without ischemic electrocardiographic changes (10.6%)[32,34] and transient bradycardia (2.6%).[32] Multiple studies have found no association between use of OCT and major procedural complications such as vasospasm, thrombi/emboli, angiographic evidence of dissections, acute vessel closure, urgent revascularization, postprocedural myocardial infarction, or death.[32–34]

Contrast

Strategies to limit the volume of contrast with OCT imaging are critical to enhance the procedural safety profile and increase the appeal of intracoronary OCT imaging by avoiding added expense and the risk of contrast nephropathy.

Table 2
Recommended power injection settings for blood clearance during OCT image acquisition

Flow Rate	Pressure	Rise	Injection Period
Left coronary: 4 mL/s Right coronary: 3 mL/s Increase by 0.5–1 mL/s in case of inadequate luminal clearing	Maximum 300 psi	Nonlinear Consider 0.3 if guide unstable with nonlinear rise	4 s Increase to 5 s if incomplete clearance at the end of run

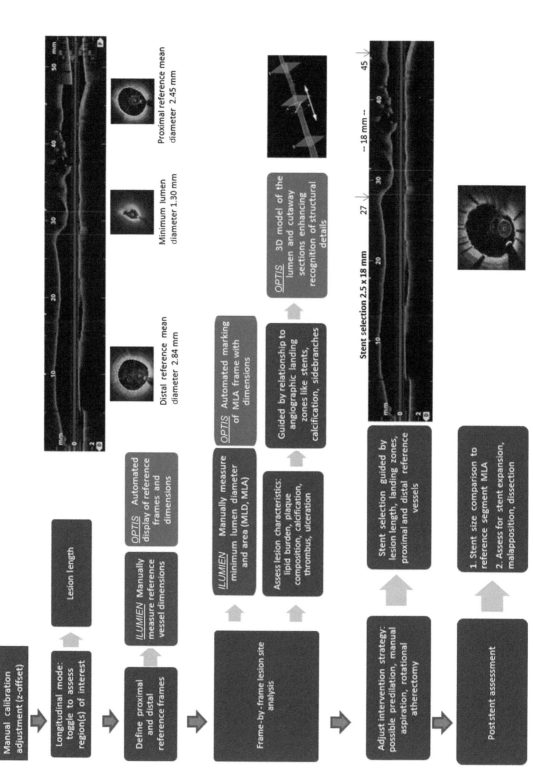

Fig. 6. Suggested protocol for in-laboratory off-line OCT analysis for coronary stent procedure guidance. 3D, 3-dimensional; MLD, minimum lumen diameter.

There are several approaches to limit contrast usage while incorporating OCT into procedural workflow. First, one may obtain both angiographic and OCT imaging simultaneously. Avoiding an additional wire-in or wire-out cineangiogram through simultaneous imaging may significantly reduce additional contrast usage.

Second, the operator should use the information gained from high-resolution OCT imaging to eliminate the need for additional angiographic views by determining the presence or absence of edge dissection, severity of untreated disease segments, and so on. Third, as noted above, some operators have successfully performed OCT imaging with 1:1 or 3:1 contrast/saline mixtures.

Fourth, an off-label approach would be to use LMD-L[35–37] as the flush agent, instead of contrast.[23,38–40] The premise of potential safety with LMD-L for FD-OCT imaging in patients with renal insufficiency is based on the fact that cumulative doses less than 1000 mL are thought to be safe, and usually no greater than 25 mL is required for flushing during OCT imaging.[21,23,37,41]

Protocol for In-Laboratory Measurements

Each operator and laboratory should develop his or her own system for off-line analysis once imaging is complete (**Fig. 6**). However there should be some protocol within the laboratory to ensure optimal technician or "super user" training, to facilitate relevant measurements quickly. The introduction of the integrated OCT system with tabletop control enhances the ability of the operator to independently and rapidly analyze the acquired imaging data set. Of the many possible measurements that can be obtained from pre-PCI imaging, most operators include lesion length assessment via the longitudinal display, distal and proximal reference lumen diameters, minimum lumen diameter (MLD), MLA at reference and lesion sites, an assessment of branch locations, and plaque characteristics. Poststent placement, routine assessment should include the MLA and MLD within the stented region compared with the reference segments, the presence of edge dissection, tissue prolapse and malapposition, and the location of stent edges relative to expected landmarks such as side branches and previous stents.

SUMMARY

Intravascular OCT imaging is a new modality for guiding interventional procedures, understanding coronary vessel architecture, and assessing neointimal growth and in-stent restenosis. The definitive clinical role for this technology is still being developed and will be guided by necessary clinical studies, but at present, interventionalists may opt to use OCT in a manner analogous to guideline-based IVUS imaging. A key factor to adopting the OCT into routine clinical practice will be adopting a procedural approach that provides the best image quality, procedural safety, and efficiency.

REFERENCES

1. Bezerra HG, Costa MA, Guagliumi G, et al. Intracoronary optical coherence tomography: a comprehensive review clinical and research applications. JACC Cardiovasc Interv 2009;2:1035–46.
2. Levine GN, Bates ER, Blankenship JC, et al. 2011 ACCF/AHA/SCAI guideline for percutaneous coronary intervention: a report of the American College of Cardiology Foundation/American Heart Association Task Force on Practice Guidelines and the Society for Cardiovascular Angiography and Interventions. Circulation 2011;124:e574–651.
3. Pijls NH, Fearon WF, Tonino PA, et al. Fractional flow reserve versus angiography for guiding percutaneous coronary intervention in patients with multivessel coronary artery disease: 2-year follow-up of the fame (fractional flow reserve versus angiography for multivessel evaluation) study. J Am Coll Cardiol 2010;56:177–84.
4. Pijls NH, van Schaardenburgh P, Manoharan G, et al. Percutaneous coronary intervention of functionally nonsignificant stenosis: 5-year follow-up of the defer study. J Am Coll Cardiol 2007;49:2105–11.
5. Briguori C, Anzuini A, Airoldi F, et al. Intravascular ultrasound criteria for the assessment of the functional significance of intermediate coronary artery stenoses and comparison with fractional flow reserve. Am J Cardiol 2001;87:136–41.
6. Koo BK, Yang HM, Doh JH, et al. Optimal intravascular ultrasound criteria and their accuracy for defining the functional significance of intermediate coronary stenoses of different locations. JACC Cardiovasc Interv 2011;4:803–11.
7. Waksman R, Legutko J, Singh J, et al. First: fractional flow reserve and intravascular ultrasound relationship study. J Am Coll Cardiol 2013;61:917–23.
8. Abizaid AS, Mintz GS, Mehran R, et al. Long-term follow-up after percutaneous transluminal coronary angioplasty was not performed based on intravascular ultrasound findings: importance of lumen dimensions. Circulation 1999;100:256–61.
9. Fedele S, Biondi-Zoccai G, Kwiatkowski P, et al. Reproducibility of coronary optical coherence

tomography for lumen and length measurements in humans (the CLI-VAR [Centro per la Lotta contro l'Infarto-VARiability] study). Am J Cardiol 2012;110:1106–12.

10. Gonzalo N, Escaned J, Alfonso F, et al. Morphometric assessment of coronary stenosis relevance with optical coherence tomography: a comparison with fractional flow reserve and intravascular ultrasound. J Am Coll Cardiol 2012;59:1080–9.

11. Lee T, Kakuta T, Yonetsu T, et al. Assessment of echo-attenuated plaque by optical coherence tomography and its impact on post-procedural creatine kinase-myocardial band elevation in elective stent implantation. JACC Cardiovasc Interv 2011;4:483–91.

12. Lee T, Yonetsu T, Koura K, et al. Impact of coronary plaque morphology assessed by optical coherence tomography on cardiac troponin elevation in patients with elective stent implantation. Circ Cardiovasc Interv 2011;4:378–86.

13. Porto I, Di Vito L, Burzotta F, et al. Predictors of periprocedural (type IVa) myocardial infarction, as assessed by frequency-domain optical coherence tomography. Circ Cardiovasc Interv 2012;5:89–96. S1–6.

14. Bouma BE, Tearney GJ, Yabushita H, et al. Evaluation of intracoronary stenting by intravascular optical coherence tomography. Heart 2003;89:317–20.

15. Guagliumi G, Sirbu V, Musumeci G, et al. Examination of the in vivo mechanisms of late drug-eluting stent thrombosis: findings from optical coherence tomography and intravascular ultrasound imaging. JACC Cardiovasc Interv 2012;5:12–20.

16. Prati F, Di Vito L, Biondi-Zoccai G, et al. Angiography alone versus angiography plus optical coherence tomography to guide decision-making during percutaneous coronary intervention: the Centro per la Lotta contro l'Infarto-Optimisation of Percutaneous Coronary Intervention (CLI-OPCI) study. EuroIntervention 2012;8:823–9.

17. McCabe JM, Croce KJ. Optical coherence tomography. Circulation 2012;126:2140–3.

18. Prati F, Regar E, Mintz GS, et al. Expert review document on methodology, terminology, and clinical applications of optical coherence tomography: physical principles, methodology of image acquisition, and clinical application for assessment of coronary arteries and atherosclerosis. Eur Heart J 2010;31:401–15.

19. Barlis P, Schmitt JM. Current and future developments in intracoronary optical coherence tomography imaging. EuroIntervention 2009;4:529–33.

20. Tearney GJ, Regar E, Akasaka T, et al. Consensus standards for acquisition, measurement, and reporting of intravascular optical coherence tomography studies: a report from the international working group for intravascular optical coherence tomography standardization and validation. J Am Coll Cardiol 2012;59:1058–72.

21. Frick K, Michael TT, Alomar M, et al. Low molecular weight dextran provides similar optical coherence tomography coronary imaging compared to radiographic contrast media. Catheter Cardiovasc Interv 2014;84:727–31.

22. Li X, Villard JW, Ouyang Y, et al. Safety and efficacy of frequency domain optical coherence tomography in pigs. EuroIntervention 2011;7:497–504.

23. Ozaki Y, Kitabata H, Tsujioka H, et al. Comparison of contrast media and low-molecular-weight dextran for frequency-domain optical coherence tomography. Circ J 2012;76:922–7.

24. Tearney GJ, Waxman S, Shishkov M, et al. Three-dimensional coronary artery microscopy by intracoronary optical frequency domain imaging. JACC Cardiovasc Imaging 2008;1:752–61.

25. Barlis P, Gonzalo N, Di Mario C, et al. A multicentre evaluation of the safety of intracoronary optical coherence tomography. EuroIntervention 2009;5:90–5.

26. Karanasos A, Ligthart J, Witberg K, et al. Optical coherence tomography: potential clinical applications. Curr Cardiovasc Imaging Rep 2012;5:206–20.

27. Prati F, Cera M, Ramazzotti V, et al. Safety and feasibility of a new non-occlusive technique for facilitated intracoronary optical coherence tomography (OCT) acquisition in various clinical and anatomical scenarios. EuroIntervention 2007;3:365–70.

28. Prati F, Cera M, Ramazzotti V, et al. From bench to bedside: a novel technique of acquiring OCT images. Circ J 2008;72:839–43.

29. Saito T, Date H, Taniguchi I, et al. Evaluation of new 4 French catheters by comparison to 6 French coronary artery images. J Invasive Cardiol 1999;11:13–20.

30. Gardiner GA Jr, Meyerovitz MF, Boxt LM, et al. Selective coronary angiography using a power injector. AJR Am J Roentgenol 1986;146:831–3.

31. Goldstein JA, Kern M, Wilson R. A novel automated injection system for angiography. J Interv Cardiol 2001;14:147–52.

32. Yoon JH, Di Vito L, Moses JW, et al. Feasibility and safety of the second-generation, frequency domain optical coherence tomography (FD-OCT): a multicenter study. J Invasive Cardiol 2012;24:206–9.

33. Takarada S, Imanishi T, Liu Y, et al. Advantage of next-generation frequency-domain optical coherence tomography compared with conventional time-domain system in the assessment of coronary lesion. Catheter Cardiovasc Interv 2010;75:202–6.

34. Imola F, Mallus MT, Ramazzotti V, et al. Safety and feasibility of frequency domain optical coherence tomography to guide decision making in

percutaneous coronary intervention. EuroIntervention 2010;6:575–81.

35. Ferraboli R, Malheiro PS, Abdulkader RC, et al. Anuric acute renal failure caused by dextran 40 administration. Ren Fail 1997;19:303–6.

36. Rothkopf DM, Chu B, Bern S, et al. The effect of dextran on microvascular thrombosis in an experimental rabbit model. Plast Reconstr Surg 1993;92:511–5.

37. Vos SC, Hage JJ, Woerdeman LA, et al. Acute renal failure during dextran-40 antithrombotic prophylaxis: report of two microsurgical cases. Ann Plast Surg 2002;48:193–6.

38. Brezinski M, Saunders K, Jesser C, et al. Index matching to improve optical coherence tomography imaging through blood. Circulation 2001;103:1999–2003.

39. Kataiwa H, Tanaka A, Kitabata H, et al. Safety and usefulness of non-occlusion image acquisition technique for optical coherence tomography. Circ J 2008;72:1536–7.

40. Kataiwa H, Tanaka A, Kitabata H, et al. Head to head comparison between the conventional balloon occlusion method and the non-occlusion method for optical coherence tomography. Int J Cardiol 2011;146:186–90.

41. Feest TG. Low molecular weight dextran: a continuing cause of acute renal failure. Br Med J 1976;2:1300.

Percutaneous Coronary Intervention Planning and Optimization with Optical Coherence Tomography

Chiara Bernelli, MD, Vasile Sirbu, MD,
Giulio Guagliumi, MD, FESC*

KEYWORDS

• Optical coherence tomography • Coronary artery disease • Percutaneous coronary interventions

---

KEY POINTS

- Optical coherence tomography (OCT) provides high-resolution, easy-to-interpret images that can help to plan and map complex percutaneous coronary interventions (PCI).
- The precise morphologic information obtained across long segments of the coronary vessels, automatic measurements, and enhanced software capabilities, make OCT more than an additional and promising intravascular tool for PCI guidance.
- Whether OCT-guided PCI leads to superior clinical outcomes versus angiography alone remains to be proven with large, prospective, randomized clinical trials.
- OCT criteria for stent optimization, based on preprocedural and postprocedural assessment, have been tested in prospective registries.
- Co-registration is a critical step-up for comprehensive integration of OCT into PCI workflow both before and after an intervention.

 Videos of OCT to diagnose nonatherosclerotic disease and OCT pull back accompany this article. http://www.interventional.theclinics.com/

INTRODUCTION: WHY OPTICAL COHERENCE TOMOGRAPHY IMAGING?

Coronary angiography is routinely used for the invasive diagnosis and treatment of coronary artery disease (CAD). For even the most experienced angiographer, however, angiography has major limitations for decision making and procedural guidance (Box 1).[1] Furthermore, the complexity of percutaneous coronary intervention (PCI) has increased significantly over time, from the original simple, isolated target lesion in the proximal coronary segment of coronary arteries to the current disease scenarios such as distal left main bifurcation and multivessel disease. In this context, intravascular imaging has emerged as a critical tool to enable physicians to deliver more precise and optimal treatment during PCI, thereby providing superior clinical outcomes.[2]

Optical coherence tomography (OCT) is a light-based imaging modality that provides tomographic views of the vessel with high axial resolution, in the range of 10 to 15 μm.[3] The

---

Disclosures: Dr C. Bernelli, report no conflicts of interest; Dr V. Sirbu reports receiving grant support from St. Jude Medical; Dr G. Guagliumi reports receiving consulting fees from Boston Scientific, St. Jude Medical and receiving grant support from St. Jude Medical, Boston Scientific and Abbott Vascular.
Interventional Cardiology Unit, Azienda Ospedaliera Papa Giovanni XXIII, Piazza OMS 1, Bergamo, 24127, Italy
* Corresponding author. Interventional Cardiology Unit, Ospedale Papa Giovanni XXIII, Piazza OMS 1, Bergamo, 24127, Italy.
E-mail address: guagliumig@gmail.com

provides a longitudinal view and lumen profile of the vessel and on-line 3-dimensional (3D) reconstruction. Based on these views, OCT promptly identifies the lesion site and severity with automatic detection of minimal lumen area (MLA) and the extension of the atherosclerotic disease. Furthermore, owing to the clarity of the acquired images, OCT does not require substantial expertise for image interpretation. After stent implantation, OCT is also more accurate than IVUS in detecting the morphologic details of suboptimal stent implantation, including underexpansion, malapposition, residual thrombus, plaque prolapse, and edge dissections.[3,10]

The key features of OCT for preprocedural use and procedural guidance are shown in **Box 2**. In follow-up stent investigations, OCT is the only imaging technique to assess precisely strut coverage and the extent of tissue growth, thereby allowing the operator to identify the underlying mechanisms of stent failure (ie, stent thrombosis and/or restenosis).

strength of OCT lays in its ability to visualize clearly the surface and subsurface of the coronary vessels with high tissue contrast, providing superb clarity of plaque composition and easier interpretation compared with intravascular ultrasound (IVUS; Table 1).[4] OCT is the only clinically available technique that can identify thin cap fibroatheroma, differentiated plaque erosion/rupture, and intraluminal thrombus with a high level of accuracy.[5–9] In addition to high-quality cross-sectional images, OCT automatically

CURRENT EVIDENCE ON OPTICAL COHERENCE TOMOGRAPHY FOR GUIDING PERCUTANEOUS CORONARY INTERVENTION

The 2014 European Society of Cardiology/European Association for Cardiothoracic Surgery Guidelines on Myocardial Revascularization state that OCT can be used in select patients to optimize stent implantation (class IIb, level of evidence C) and to assess the mechanisms related to stent failure (class IIa, level of evidence C).[11]

Table 1
Advantages and limits of intravascular imaging modalities

	Advantages	Disadvantages
IVUS	Good depth of penetration	Limited axial resolution (>100 µm)
	Tomographic view without blood removal	Low speed in pullback
	Detection of remodeling and plaque mass	Limits in presence of thrombus and calcium
	Details on plaque composition (IVUS-VH)	Not easy to be interpreted
OCT	High axial resolution images ($\cong$10 µm)	Requires displacement of blood
	High rate of data acquisition	Limited depth of penetration
	Rapid to perform Easy to be interpreted	Lot of details, relative value to be clinically proved
	High quality longitudinal view	Need of additionally contrast
	3D-vessel reconstruction	
	Detection of thrombus, thin cap fibroatheroma, culprit plaques rupture, causes of stent failure	

Abbreviations: IVUS, intravascular ultrasound; OCT, optical coherence tomography.

According to the 2013 European Society of Cardiology Guidelines on the Management of Stable CAD, OCT can be considered to further characterize the target lesions (class IIb, level of evidence B) and to improve stent deployment (class IIb, level of evidence B).[12] A recent Society of Cardiovascular Angiography and Interventions Consensus Statement recommended that OCT is "probably beneficial" to determine optimal stent placement (sizing, apposition, and lack of edge dissection) and "possibly beneficial" for assessing plaque morphology.[13]

To date, there are no prospective, randomized trials assessing the role of OCT for guiding PCI. However, several reports have shown the potential of OCT to support clinical decision making in PCI.[14–18] In pilot study of 90 patients undergoing PCI with OCT, OCT findings led to additional interventions in 32% (eg, additional balloon dilatation and stenting); the 6-month event-free survival rate was 98%.[14] Stefano and colleagues[15] reported a series of 150 consecutive patients in whom OCT was used for pre-PCI evaluation and/or stent optimization. Pre-PCI OCT prompted changes in the original angiography-guided strategy in 82% of the cases. Almost one-half of the angiographically planned stent length, one-quarter of stent diameters, and more than one-half of post-dilation balloon diameters were changed based on OCT measures. The use of OCT after PCI led to further interventions in 55% of the target vessels, mostly with additional balloon dilations to correct stent underexpansion or malapposition, or with additional stent implantation to treat edge dissection. In a study of 108 patients undergoing OCT-guided coronary stenting, the procedure was deferred based on OCT findings in 19.1% of cases and resulted in further interventions in 34%.[16]

Prati and colleagues[17] compared the 1-year clinical outcomes in 335 patients with OCT guidance with a matched control group undergoing PCI with angiographic guidance alone. The protocol provided several treatment recommendations based on OCT findings: (1) edge dissections (width >200 μm) with reference lumen narrowing (lumen area <4 mm²) were treated with additional stenting; (2) stent underexpansion (in-stent MLA ≤90% of the average reference lumen area, or MLA ≤100% of the lowest lumen area of the reference segments) had further dilation with a noncompliant balloon of the same size at 18 atm or greater, or with a semicompliant balloon with a diameter 0.25 mm larger, at 14 atm or greater; (3) stent malapposition at a distance of greater than 200 μm required further dilation of the implanted stent with a noncompliant or semicompliant balloon; and (4) residual intraluminal thrombus after stenting was further dilated with a noncompliant or semicompliant balloon of the same diameter, for 60 seconds. OCT identified suboptimal features requiring additional interventions in 35% of cases. On unadjusted analysis, the OCT group had a significantly lower 1-year risk of cardiac death (1.2% vs 4.5%; $P = .01$), cardiac death or myocardial infarction (MI; 6.6% vs 13%; $P = .006$), and the composite of cardiac death, MI, or repeat revascularization (9.6% vs 14.8%; $P = .044$) compared with angiographic guidance alone. After adjustments by multivariate and propensity score–adjusted analysis, OCT-guided PCI was associated with a lower risk of cardiac death or MI (odds ratio, 0.49; 95% CI, 0.25–0.96; $P = .037$). At a technical level, the difference between the treatment groups was driven mainly by the elimination of all potential adverse OCT features.[18] Therefore, these studies suggest that OCT has potential clinical benefit in the planning and mapping PCI procedures to optimize the results of stent implantation.

ESSENTIAL COMPONENTS FOR USING OPTICAL COHERENCE TOMOGRAPHY TO GUIDE PERCUTANEOUS CORONARY INTERVENTION

OCT can be performed and interpreted easily in the majority of clinical settings (Fig. 1). To obtain high-quality tissue contrast, it is necessary to appropriately select and engage the guiding catheter, correctly position the OCT imaging

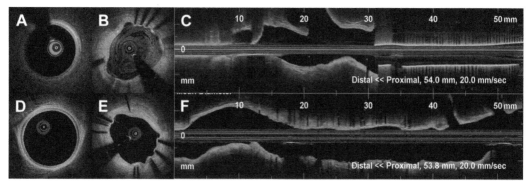

Fig. 1. Necessary conditions for adequate imaging acquisition. (A) Inadequate purging of optical coherence tomography (OCT) catheter, resulting in image attenuation. (B) Image attenuation owing to inadequate contrast flushing and incomplete clearance of blood from the vessel lumen. (C) Insufficient imaging of the length of the vessel owing to inappropriate positioning of the imaging element, leading to excessive length of the guiding catheter within the OCT run (from 30 mm up to 50 mm). (D, E) Cross-sections. (F; long view) OCT image obtained with proper guide position, imaging catheter position, and vessel flushing.

catheter across the region of interest, and adequately flush with contrast. A quick test injection before the pullback is usually valuable to ensure adequate flushing and minimize wasted contrast if guide engagement is insufficient. In general, OCT should be performed as a part of the diagnostic procedure because it provides crucial information for the operator to decide and plan the intervention (Box 3). Table 2 summarizes the application of OCT compared with IVUS in clinical practice.

The latest generation OCT systems provide automatic lumen profile contour through a frame-by-frame detection border algorithm. The lumen profile immediately available at the end of the pullback automatically displays the MLA

and minimal lumen diameter, the percentage of area of stenosis, and the normal reference segments (Fig. 2) across the entire vessel. Lumen dimensions, extension of vessel disease, and vessel tapering are of paramount importance for planning PCI. The reproducibility of lumen area and length measurements obtained by OCT has been demonstrated repeatedly.[19–22] In the prospective multicenter study, OPUS-CLASS (OCT Compared With IVUS in a Coronary Lesion Assessment) Fourier domain-OCT was compared with quantitative coronary angiography and IVUS in 100 consecutive patients to assess the relative accuracy of MLA and minimal lumen diameter measurements.[21] OCT underestimated the MLA by approximately 9% compared with IVUS, but OCT was significantly more accurate in measuring the actual phantom lumen area ($P<.001$), suggesting that Fourier domain -OCT is superior with respect to real measurements. Finally, the high density of imaging frames obtained with OCT enables high-quality 3D reconstruction that, combined with cross-sectional and longitudinal views, allows a more complete visualization of complex anatomy, including ostia, bifurcations, side branches, and stent geometry.

USE OF OPTICAL COHERENCE TOMOGRAPHY IN CLINICAL PRACTICE

OCT may be used at different time points during cardiac catheterization (Box 4): (1) before intervention to define or to confirm the diagnosis of severe CAD and to identify the need for subsequent PCI; (2) during the PCI procedure to plan and guide the intervention step by step;

Box 3
When to use optical coherence tomography imaging

High-risk patient subsets

   Acute coronary syndrome

   Patients with stent thrombosis and in-stent restenosis

   Diabetes mellitus

High-risk lesion subsets

   Bifurcations (including distal left main disease)

   Small vessels

   Long lesions

   Diffuse disease

   Vessel tapering

Table 2
A user's guide to OCT application in clinical practice

Recommendations for IVUS[a]	Class (LOE)[a]	Applicability of OCT	Advantage of OCT	Disadvantage of OCT
I. Assessment of distal left main	II a (B)	No if ostial	High spatial resolution (3D) but vision must be ameliorated	Large vessel size may limit visualization No studies available
II. Guidance of coronary stent implantation	II b (B)	Yes	Highly reproducible vessel measurements (long view, automatic measures) aid stent length and diameter selection Risk stratification for periprocedural myocardial infarction (complex lesions and patients) More commonly identifies segment of malapposition and edge dissections	Not applicable in ostial left main or ostial right coronary artery No evidence that OCT-guided PCI improves clinical outcomes (criteria TBD, possible) Contrast use, extra time
III. Determine the mechanism of stent restenosis/ stent thrombosis	II a/II b (C)	Yes	Accurate identification of strut malapposition, undererxpansion, edge dissections, stent fracture, and in-stent neoatherosclerosis Strut coverage	Requires further study (eg, "PREvention of Stent Thrombosis by an Interdisciplinary Global European effort" PRESTIGE available in 2015)
IV. Exclude donor coronary artery disease and detect rapidly progressive cardiac allograft vasculopathy 4–6 wk and 1 y after cardiac transplantation	II a (B)	Preliminary	Tissue characterization Intimal media thickness measurements: similar to IVUS Higher resolution allows more sensitive measure of early intimal thickening.	Clinical predictive; value uncertain (personalized immunotherapy)

Abbreviations: IVUS, intravascular ultrasound; LOE, level of evidence; OCT, optical coherence tomography; PCI, Percutaneous Coronary Intervention; TBD, to be determined.

[a] Recommendations for IVUS and class (LOE) adapted from 2011 American College of Cardiology Foundation/ American Heart Association/Society of Cardiac Angiography Interventions Guidelines for IVUS.

Adapted from Lopez JJ, Arain SA, Madder R, et al. Techniques and best practices for optical coherence tomography: a practical manual for interventional cardiologists. Catheter Cardiovasc Interv 2014;84:687–99.

and (3) after PCI, to assess PCI and stent results and to optimize the stent implantation as needed.

Optical Coherence Tomography After Diagnostic Angiography and Before Intervention

Diagnosis and characterization of coronary atherosclerosis

OCT has been proved to be highly accurate in characterizing and differentiating early from advanced coronary vessel pathology.[3] In addition, OCT is able to identify morphologic characteristics of plaques at risk of rupture (vulnerable plaques), including fibrous cap thickness, the presence of microvessels, macrophage infiltration toward the cap, and thrombus formation.[6,7,23–27] All of these features make OCT an invaluable imaging tool for in vivo characterization of plaque types, components, and mechanisms of disease progression (Fig. 3).

Nonatherosclerotic coronary artery disease

Although most lesions identified on angiography are atherosclerotic in origin, some reduction of the coronary lumen results from different mechanisms. In uncertain clinical scenarios, OCT may orient the diagnosis and treatment toward

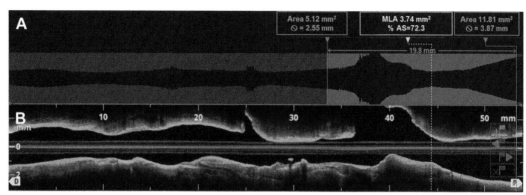

Fig. 2. Lumen profile. (A) Example of longitudinal reconstruction of the target vessel by automated border detection for the assessment of lesion length and severity. Real-time measurements of the reference vessel areas, reference vessel diameters, and lesion length are displayed in blue, and the minimal luminal diameter and area in yellow. (B) Optical coherence tomography longitudinal view and site. Φ, mean diameter; AS, area stenosis; MLA, minimal lumen area.

nonatherosclerotic CAD, including spontaneous coronary artery dissection and immune-mediated microvascular disease, such as scleroderma (Fig. 4, Video 1).[28,29]

Unclear and challenging situations
OCT may help in clarifying unclear lesions with angiographic haziness, particularly in the case of acute coronary syndrome (Fig. 5). Under

---

Box 4
OCT for decision making and in planning PCI in the catheterization laboratory

Preintervention (diagnostic and planning intervention's purposes)

    Assessment of unclear lesion(s)

    Qualitative and quantitative assessment of the vessel and lesion/s

    Planning intervention and PCI technique (bifurcations including distal left main)

    Optimal balloon size, length, type

    Lesion preparation (cutting balloon, rotablator, BVS implantation)

Procedural guidance and PCI optimization

    Identification of landing zone

    Vessel tapering

    Identification of additional pretreatment before stent implantation

    Selection of optimal stent diameter and length

    Additional stent implantation

    Evaluation of MLA/MSA, stent expansion (additional balloon dilatation with higher pressure/larger balloons)

    Edge dissection/s

    Stent malapposition

    Stent distortion (eg, additional final kissing balloon in bifurcations)

Long-term assessment of PCI results

    Level and possible maturity of stent coverage

    Assessment of mechanisms related and associated with stent failure (eg, stent thrombosis, in-stent restenosis, stent fracture)

    Accurate planning and customized treatment of stent failure

Abbreviations: BVS, bioresorbable vascular scaffold; MLA, minimal lumen area; MSA, minimal stent area; OCT, optical coherence tomography; PCI, percutaneous coronary intervention.

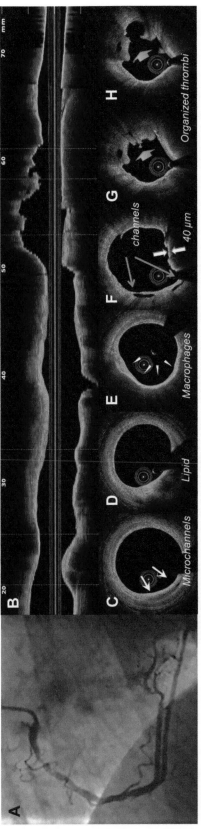

Fig. 3. Optical coherence tomography (OCT) evaluation of culprit and distal sites in non–ST-elevation acute coronary syndrome. (A), Coronary angiography demonstrates a hazy appearing lesion within the proximal right coronary artery. (B) Longitudinal view of the culprit vessel (75 mm pullback length) demonstrating the culprit site with an irregular luminal border and protruding material (see marker 45–65) as well as a remote site in the mid-to-distal segment with important plaque burden (see marker 20–40). (C–E) Cross-sectional images of the remote site within the mid-to-distal segment demonstrating OCT characteristics of vulnerable plaque: microchannels (white arrows in C), lipid-rich plaque (from 6 to 9 o'clock in D), and foamy macrophage accumulations (white arrowheads in E). (F–H) Cross-sectional images from the culprit site demonstrating the presence of channels (blue arrows in F), thin-capped fibroatheroma (white arrows in F), and organized thrombi (blue arrow in G, H).

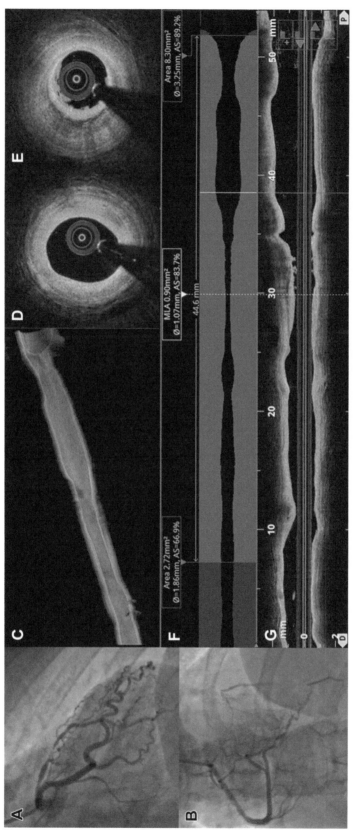

Fig. 4. Optical coherence tomography (OCT) to diagnose nonatherosclerotic disease: scleroderma. (A) Coronary angiography of the left anterior descending artery demonstrates a long, subtotal occlusion. (B) Coronary angiography of the right coronary artery demonstrates collaterals to the distal and mid left anterior descending. (C–G) OCT of the left anterior descending demonstrates diffuse, intimal medial thickening, a finding suggestive of a fibrotic process rather than de novo atherosclerosis. (C) Three-dimensional reconstruction of OCT pullback of the left anterior descending artery. (D, E) Cross-sections at the site of minimal luminal area demonstrating the absence of atherosclerotic plaque and the presence of a fibrotic process suggestive of autoimmune origin. (F) Lumen profile tool providing information about the severity of the stenosis. (G) Longitudinal reconstruction providing information regarding the extent of the pathology. AS, area stenosis; MLA, minimal lumen area.

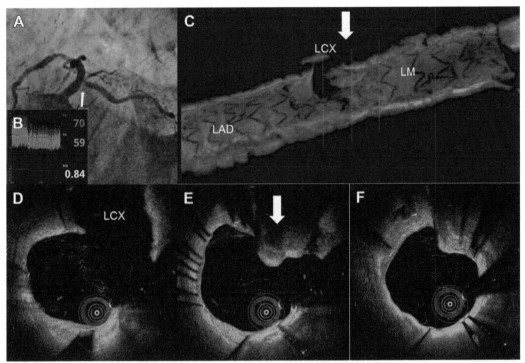

Fig. 5. Optical coherence tomography (OCT) evaluation of an angiographically hazy lesion. (A) Coronary angiography demonstrates a hazy lesion within the ostium of the left circumflex artery. (B) Fractional flow reserve (FFR) performed on the left circumflex artery was negative. (C) Three-dimensional reconstruction provides information regarding the relationship and position of a calcium spicule at the left main bifurcation. (D–F) Consecutive OCT cross-sections at the level of distal left main and circumflex ostium show the hazy imaging on angiography was owing to a heavy calcific spicule (*arrow*) protruding into the lumen, with distortion of the cell geometry (see 3D view in C). LAD, left anterior descending; LCX, left circumflex; LM, left main.

these circumstances, the decision to proceed with treatment depends not only from the accurate measurement of the MLA (which is difficult in the presence of angiographic haziness), but also from morphologic plaque features. OCT can be used to differentiate culprit plaque with thrombus deposition compared with protruding calcium (**Fig. 6**). Misinterpretation of the culprit

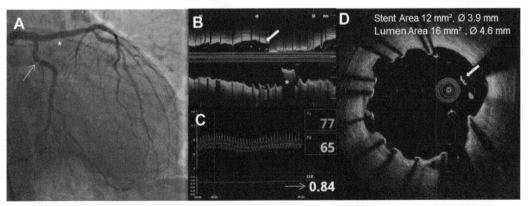

Fig. 6. Combined use of optical coherence tomography (OCT) and fractional flow reserve for culprit lesion identification. (A) Coronary angiography of a patient with a recurrence of acute coronary syndrome demonstrates an area of haziness inside a previously implanted everolimus-eluting stent within the left anterior descending artery (*asterisk*), and a tight-appearing, focal stenosis within the mid left circumflex artery (*arrow*). (B) OCT longitudinal view of the left anterior descending shows the thrombotic nature of the hazy lesion (*asterisk*) and clusters of uncovered struts (*arrow*). (C) Fractional flow reserve performed on the left circumflex artery was negative, thus excluding this as the culprit lesion. (D) Close review of OCT cross-section reveals clusters of uncovered and malapposed stent struts (*arrow*).

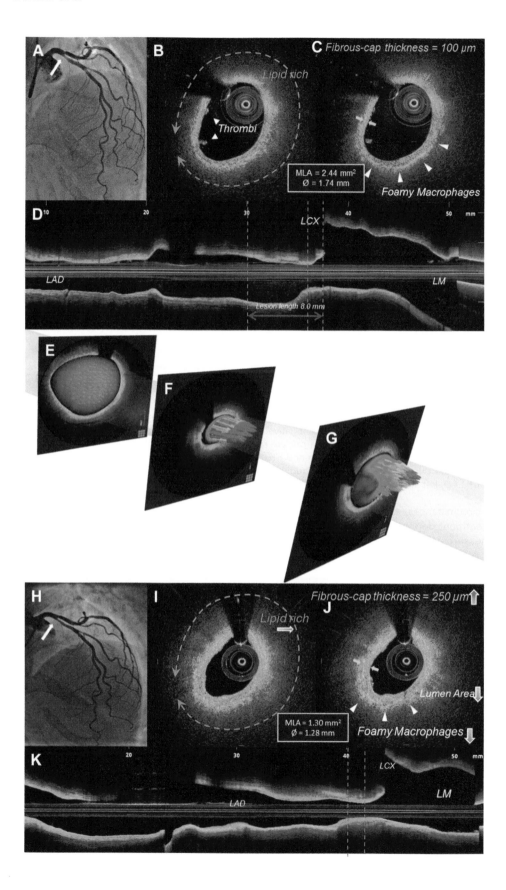

lesion could be the cause of additional early adverse ischemic events in patients with acute coronary syndrome. The presence of angiographic haziness after stent implantation may also be owing to multiple causes and mechanisms: for example, remaining soft plaque adjacent to the stent, remnants of a preexisting thrombus, or a stent edge dissection.

Prediction of lesion progression and vulnerability

OCT may help to identify lesions that might be at high risk of progression and future adverse events. Of particular interest is the ability of OCT to detect lipid-rich thin cap fibroatheroma combined with microvessels and foamy macrophages, the latter recognized by the accumulation of bright spots with sharp signal attenuation near the luminal border. Combined angiographic and OCT images with additional mathematic computation of flow velocity and shear stress may possibly allow a better prediction of plaque evolution (Fig. 7).

Optical Coherence Tomography for Planning Percutaneous Coronary Interventions
Automatic border detection, fibrous cap thickness, and landing zones

Although fractional flow reserve is the gold standard for assessing the functional significance of angiographically intermediate lesions, OCT has a complementary role in mapping the vessel pathology (lesion type, extension, geometry, and branch relationship) that may help in guiding the PCI procedure (Fig. 8).[30] The accurate identification of plaque components and normal reference segments by means of OCT are key features to improve PCI.[3] These OCT findings may suggest how to treat the lesion and where to land the stent to avoid immediate ischemic complications, for example, direct stenting without embolic protection in presence of a thick cap fibroatheroma (Fig. 9). The identification of normal or "less diseased" reference vessel for accurate stent placement is of pivotal importance in PCI (Fig. 10). Landing a stent over a thin cap fibroatheroma has been associated independently with the occurrence of periprocedural MI, whereas disruption of such areas may lead to increased risk of neoatherosclerosis and late stent thrombosis, as suggested by OCT and pathologic studies.[31,32] It has also been demonstrated that the frequency of no-reflow phenomenon increases according to the lipid content of the plaque and the thinning of the cap as assessed by OCT.[33] In addition, plaque composition at the stent edges has been associated with the occurrence of stent dissections and future restenosis.[34,35] Avoidance of landing a stent edge within a TFCA or calcified plaque reduces the rate of edge dissections.[36]

Calcification

The continuous increase in age of patients presenting with CAD, combined with the substantial impact of comorbidities (diabetes, renal failure) and the limited value of angiography in detecting vessel calcification, suggest that OCT may be the best imaging technique for PCI guidance in the presence of calcium. Light has the ability to penetrate calcium fully (a major limitation of ultrasonography), to delineate its border, and to assess the circumferential and axial extent at a very high level of accuracy (Fig. 11).[37] The presence, depth, and circumferential extent of calcification can affect negatively the results of PCI (Fig. 12).[38,39] In the case of an extensive calcification lesion undetected by angiography, OCT imaging may suggest avoiding direct stenting or the use of bioresorbable vascular scaffolds (BVS), and instead using a scoring balloon and/or a rotational atherectomy of adequate burr size for lesion preparation. The ability of OCT to precisely assess calcium accumulation and

Fig. 7. Plaque features conditioning lesion progression. (*A*) Coronary angiography demonstrates an indeterminate stenosis of the proximal left anterior descending (LAD) with a hazy appearance (*arrow*). (*B*) Optical coherence tomography (OCT) cross-section at the level of the stenosis demonstrates lipid-rich plaque and microthrombi (*arrowheads*). (*C*) OCT cross-section of the same segment shows foamy macrophage accumulations (*arrowheads*) within the cap of the atheroma (*arrows*) close to the lumen. (*D*) Longitudinal reconstruction demonstrates that the stenosis is caused by a lipid-rich plaque that extends from distal segment of the left main into the proximal segment of the left anterior descending. (*E–G*) Fluid dynamics study showing blood velocity vectors overlapped on OCT image showing normal velocities at the proximal reference site (*E*), acceleration at site of minimal luminal area (*F*) and recirculation flows at the distal reference vessel (*G*). (*H*) Coronary angiography after 2 months of optimal medial therapy revealing progression of the proximal left anterior descending stenosis (*arrow*). (*I, J*) Cross-sections showing maintenance of the lipid arc (*I, arrow*), increase in cap thickness (*J, arrow*), reduction of foamy macrophages (*arrowheads*), and reduction of minimal luminal area. (*K*) Longitudinal reconstruction showing lesion extension. LCX, Left circumflex; LM, left main; MLA, minimal lumen area.

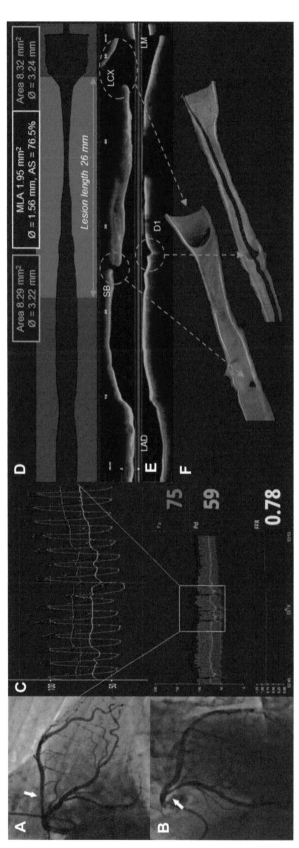

Fig. 8. Optical coherence tomography for PCI planning. (A, B) Coronary angiography of a lesion of intermediate severity within the proximal segment of the left anterior descending artery (arrows). (C) Fractional flow reserve evaluation demonstrated reduced ratio of mean distal pressure to proximal pressure during maximal hyperemia, consistent with a physiologically important stenosis (fractional flow reserve = 0.78). (D–F) Lumen profile, longitudinal reconstruction and 3-dimensional (3D) view. (D) Lumen profile tool identifies the lesion site, which has a 77% area stenosis, a lesion length of 26 mm, and proximal and distal reference vessel diameters of 3.24 and 3.22 mm, respectively, informing the appropriate stent selection. (F) Three-dimensional reconstruction highlights the relationship of the lesion to the left circumflex ostium and major left anterior descending side branches. AS, area stenosis; D1, first diagonal branch; LAD, left anterior descending; LCX, left circumflex; LM, left main; MLA, minimal lumen area; SB, septal branch.

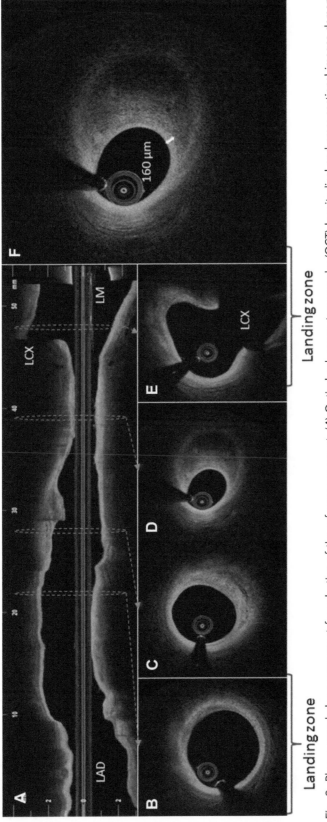

Fig. 9. Plaque morphology assessment for selection of the reference segment. (A) Optical coherence tomography (OCT) longitudinal and cross-sectional images demonstrating an eccentric, lipid-rich plaque involving the ostium of the left anterior descending. (B) OCT cross-section displaying distal "normal" reference segment. (C) Cross-section presenting adjacent to the segment of the minimal luminal area. (D) Cross-section of the site of minimal luminal area. (E) Cross-section showing proximal "normal" reference segment. (F), Zoom on the site of minimal luminal area demonstrating a thick fibrous cap atheroma (minimum fibrous cap thickness = 160 μm), (arrow) indicated a low risk of distal embolization associated with percutaneous coronary intervention. LAD, left anterior descending; LCX, left circumflex; LM, left main.

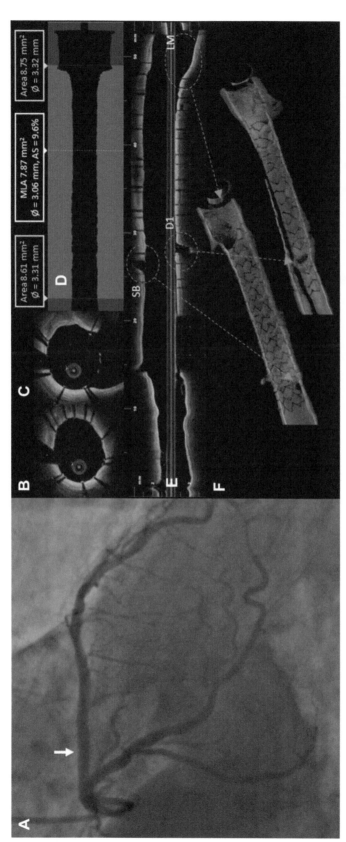

Fig. 10. Optical coherence tomography (OCT) to control acute result of stent implantation. (A) Coronary angiography after implantation of a drug-eluting stent (DES) within the ostium of the LAD (arrow). (B) OCT cross-section showing uniform stent expansion. (C) OCT cross-section of the proximal stent edge, which was placed just at the ostium of LAD. (D) Post-PCI lumen profile demonstrates uniform stent expansion with minimum stent area of 7.9 mm². (E) Longitudinal view confirms uniform stent expansion without edge dissection. (F) Three-dimensional OCT reconstruction confirms perfect coverage of the ostial lesion with minimum strut protrusion into the left main bifurcation. D1, first diagonal; LM, left main; MLA, minimal lumen area; SB, septal branch.

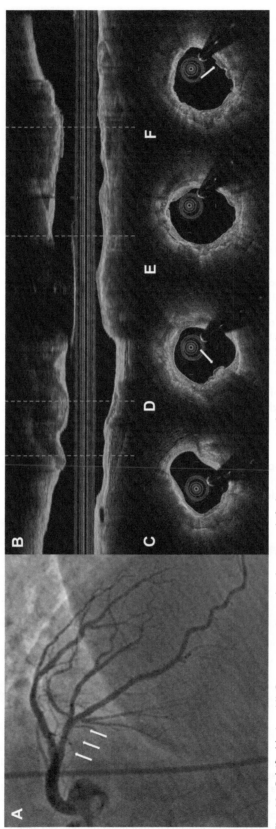

Fig. 11. Calcified lesion. (A) Coronary angiography showing calcific lesion (arrows) of the proximal left anterior descending artery. (B) Longitudinal reconstruction showing extension of heavy calcification of the proximal left anterior descending. (C–F) Optical coherence tomography cross-sections showing 360° circumferential extension of the calcified lesion, with a calcium spicule protruding into the coronary lumen (arrow).

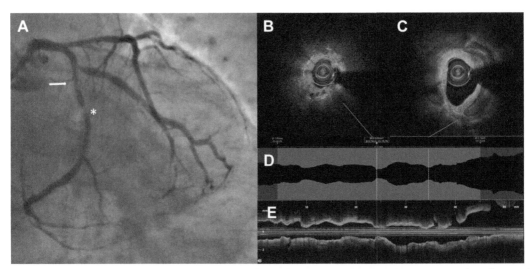

Fig. 12. Assessment of plaque morphology before PCI. (A) Coronary angiography demonstrates a hazy lesion of intermediate severity in the proximal left circumflex (*arrow*) and an angiographically significant lesion (*asterisk*) within the mid left circumflex. (B) Optical coherence tomography (OCT) cross-section at the level of the angiographically significant stenosis demonstrates a morphologic pattern consistent with fibrotic plaque. (C) OCT cross-section at the level of the hazy intermediate stenosis demonstrates morphology consistent with a heavy, calcific plaque with circumferential extension. (D) Lumen profile tool provides an immediate calculation of lesion severity and visualization of the extent of pathology. (E) Longitudinal reconstruction demonstrates diffuse atherosclerotic involvement within the region of interest.

distribution (arc of circumference) within the vessel wall may significantly impact the final result of PCI (Fig. 13).

Vessel tapering
The sudden changes in coronary lumen dimensions that can be seen on angiography after the take off of major side branches (vessel tapering) often represents a challenge for correct stent selection and full stent apposition to the vessel wall. Vessel tapering is a normal phenomenon, especially in within the left coronary arteries. It must be considered when approaching a long coronary diseased segment (especially in the left anterior descending artery) and/or in the presence of a main vessel lesion

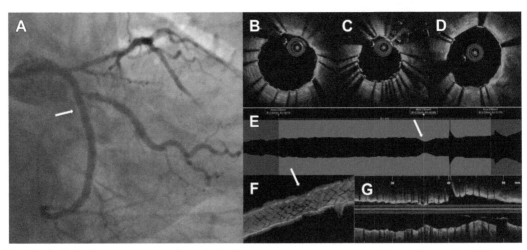

Fig. 13. Optical coherence tomography analysis of acute percutaneous coronary intervention results. (A) Coronary angiography after drug-eluting stent implantation within the left circumflex (*arrow*). (B–D) Complete stent apposition and symmetric geometry of the implanted stent. (C) Stent underexpansion at the level of the calcified lesion. (E) Lumen profile and longitudinal view demonstrates 40% residual stenosis within the stented segment (*arrow*). (F) Three-dimensional reconstruction demonstrates "crowded" strut area corresponding with the stent underexpansion (*arrow*). (G) Longitudinal OCT resonstruction showing no stent malapposition and wide access to the side branch.

extending across a large side branch. OCT imaging that assesses long segments of coronary arteries and displays an automatic lumen profile can detect easily exaggerated vessel tapering, suggesting the most appropriate stent selection (**Fig. 14**). After stent implantation, accurate visualization and quantification of stent and vessel dimensions provided by OCT as well as the 3D reconstruction can detect incomplete stent expansion, malapposition, and distortion, thereby guiding and mapping any additional intervention for stent optimization (**Fig. 15**).

Acute coronary syndromes and primary percutaneous coronary intervention

OCT is useful to provide insights into the pathophysiology of acute coronary syndrome, differentiating between plaque rupture/erosion and calcified nodules.[3] In addition, OCT gives accurate information on plaque composition, fibrous cap thickness, and the presence of thrombus, microvessels and foamy macrophages that characterize advanced plaque at high risk for future adverse events.[40–42] The prompt identification of these elements contributes to the ultimate therapeutic approach, orienting periprocedural decisions and postprocedural PCI optimization. OCT can be safely performed in patients with ST-segment elevation MI. However, in the case of complete vessel occlusion (ie, Thrombolysis In Myocardial Infarction [TIMI] 0–1 flow), restoration of vessel patency with thrombectomy needs to be obtained before the OCT pullback to ensure adequate clearing of the vessel lumen during contrast injection so that adequate images can be obtained. The effectiveness of thrombus removal and any further need for thrombus aspiration can be easily identified by OCT. Furthermore, the high-resolution longitudinal view and 3D reconstruction can display the relationship between the remaining thrombus and the location of major side branches (**Fig. 16**). The remaining thrombus may also increase the risk of subsequent stent failure (eg, stent thrombosis, late

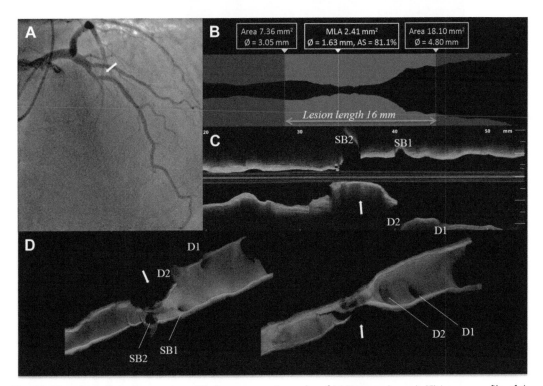

Fig. 14. Vessel tapering phenomenon. (*A*) Coronary angiography of LAD artery (*arrow*). (*B*) Lumen profile of the optical coherence tomography imaging pullback within the LAD confirms the presence of substantial vessel tapering between proximal and distal reference segments (mean proximal diameter, 4.8 mm vs mean distal diameter, 3.1 mm). (*C*) Longitudinal reconstruction shows that the stenosis is caused by a lipid-rich plaque (*arrow*) involving the second diagonal and second septal branches. (*D*) Three-dimensional view provides orientation of the spatial distribution of the plaque, and its relation to the take-off of the side branches (*arrow*). Φ, mean diameter; D1, D2, diagonal branches; LAD, left anterior descending artery; SB1, SB2, septal branches.

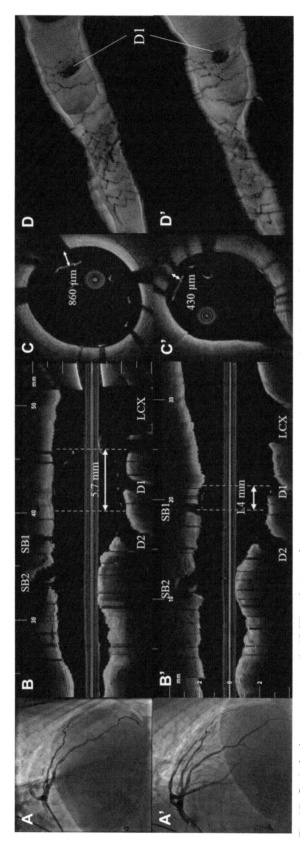

Fig. 15. Optical coherence tomography (OCT) evaluation of percutaneous coronary intervention result in the setting of substantial vessel tapering. (A) Coronary angiography showing immediate result of drug-eluting stent implantation. (B) OCT pullback in LAD reveals a long segment of stent malapposition (5.7 mm) owing to substantial discrepancy in vessel diameter between the distal and proximal reference segments. (C) Cross-section at the proximal edge shows a distance of 860 μm between stent strut and vessel wall. (D) Three-dimensional reconstruction orientates the spatial distribution of the stent and shows distortion of stent geometry owing to large diameter post-dilatation balloon inflation. (A′)- Coronary angiography shows immediate result of drug-eluting implantation. (B′) OCT pullback in LAD reveals reduction in the length of the malapposed segment (1.4 mm) after repeated post dilatations with larger balloons. (C′) Cross-section at the proximal edge demonstrates a reduced distance (430 μm) between stent strut and vessel wall. (D′) Three-dimensional reconstruction orientates the spatial distribution of the stent and shows further distortion of stent geometry owing to post dilatation with larger balloons. D1, D2, first and second diagonal branches; LAD, left anterior descending artery; LCX, left circumflex artery; SB1, SB2, first and second septal branches.

acquired incomplete stent apposition owing to clot reabsorption, and neoatherosclerosis). In addition, enhanced vessel constriction makes it difficult to select the appropriate stent sizing and length.[43–46] In this setting, stent size and length should be selected based on accurate lumen assessment by OCT. Stent underexpansion, malapposition, edge dissection, and complete coverage of the culprit lesion should also be evaluated and corrected to optimize the results of primary PCI (Fig. 17).

Bifurcation lesions

The complexity in treating bifurcation lesions arises from both anatomic and flow characteristics. Plaque distribution, carina geometry, and the bifurcation angle have a great impact on PCI strategy selection and rate of side branch occlusion after stenting. To optimize the acute results of stent implantation and minimize the risk for side branch occlusion and/or late stent failure, detailed information on the lesion involving the bifurcation should be collected before and after the treatment. Atheroma distribution and type of carina are key information for planning PCI strategy and minimize the risk of side branch occlusion owing to the carina/plaque shift. In line with IVUS data, OCT demonstrates frequently that the plaque accumulates less toward the flow divider region,

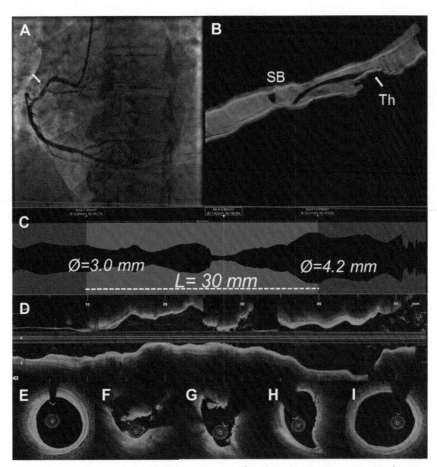

Fig. 16. Optical coherence tomography (OCT) assessment after thrombus aspiration in ST-elevation myocardial infarction. (A) Coronary angiography after thrombus aspiration of a thrombotic lesion in the proximal segment of right coronary artery (arrow). (B) Three-dimensional OCT reconstruction demonstrates a large amount of residual thrombus protruding into the lumen (arrow). (C) Lumen profile confirms significant vessel tapering from proximal to distal to the lesion. (D) Longitudinal OCT reconstruction showing distribution of the atherosclerotic pathology within the coronary artery. (E, I) "Normal" reference segments for planning where to land with the stent were selected at sites of minimum plaque burden and fibrotic plaque characteristics. (F–H, cross-sections of culprit lesion, demonstrating thin cap fibroatheroma and eroded plaques). Th, thrombus.

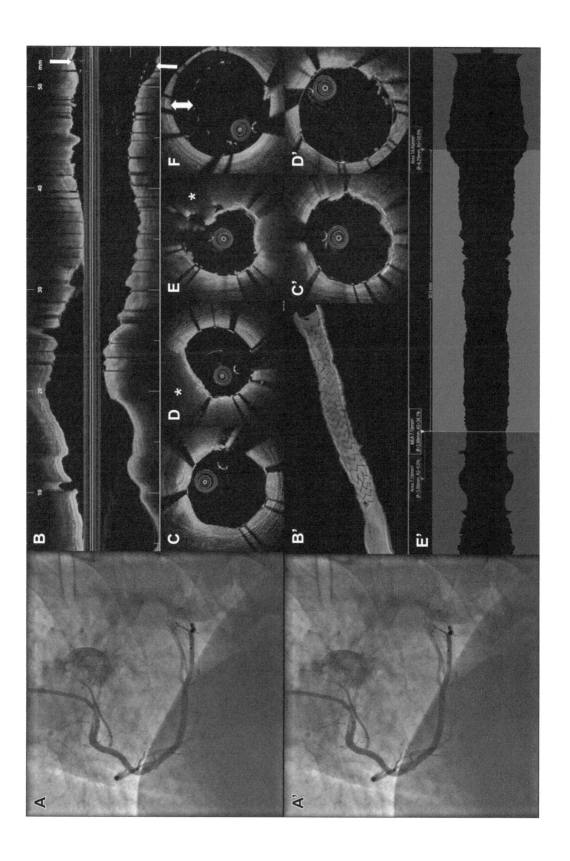

compared with the opposite wall of the bifurcation, where low shear area is prevalent (Fig. 18).[47] In addition, the anatomic type of carina and degree of plaque involvement can help to anticipate side branch obstruction after provisional stent implantation. Even if spared from lesion involvement, an elongated carina may cause obstruction of the side branch ostium after stent implantation in the main vessel.[48] This morphology ("spikey" or "eyebrow" carina) can be easily detected by preintervention OCT, particularly on the high-resolution longitudinal view and the 3D reconstruction (Fig. 19).[49–52] The presence of an "eyebrow" carina should lead the operator to protect the side branch ostium (ie, with a second coronary wire), even in absence of ostial pathology. OCT can guide a more accurate wire crossing if rewiring of the stent implanted in the main vessel is required to get access to the side branch ostium, thereby avoiding stent distortion.

Left main disease

OCT imaging enables a quick evaluation of shaft and distal bifurcation left main disease. With the exception of ostial lesions, OCT can be used to precisely assess plaque distribution and to evaluate the left main lumen area with similar accuracy compared with IVUS.[53] Furthermore, OCT is superior to IVUS in visualizing intraluminal thrombus, which is an additional risk factor in this setting. In unprotected left main PCI, preprocedural OCT assessment is essential to evaluate (1) the extension of the disease into the left anterior descending and/or left circumflex arteries, (2) plaque type, (3) the anatomic type of carina and the degree of lesion involvement, and (4) the magnitude of the size differential between the left main and the distal landing zone (ie, degree of vessel tapering; Fig. 20). After intervention, OCT detects with greater accuracy than IVUS the presence of dissection, stent malapposition, underexpansionm and size mismatch.[53] Dense jailing of the ostia,

geographic miss, and longitudinal compression of stents can be also identified on OCT. Overall, these are essential data that may guide the optimization of unprotected left main PCI, eliminating predisposing features for stent thrombosis that could be particularly devastating at this location in the coronary tree (Fig. 21).

Implantation of bioresorbable vascular scaffolds

The main advantages of BVS are temporary vascular scaffolding combined with drug delivery capability. BVS may acts as a "vascular restoration therapy" that reestablishes in a reasonable time vessel physiology and anatomy. OCT had a major role in the development of BVS technology and in furnishing proof of the scaffold's biological and mechanical characteristics.[54] Serial OCT assessment of the vascular response after BVS implantation demonstrated that scaffold dimensions progressively increase, with unchanged lumen area between 1 and 3 years, and complete strut reabsorption at 3 to 5 years after implantation. Although metallic stent struts are not penetrated by the light beam (causing significant signal attenuation), light is not attenuated by the polymeric struts of BVS and therefore they seem to be transparent on OCT imaging, allowing for the full visualization of the vessel structure behind the scaffold (Fig. 22). BVS compared with current DES has a larger crossing profile (1.4–1.5 mm), greater strut thickness (≈ 160 μm), and less radial force, especially when confronted with the most advanced, calcified, and complex lesions. Different plaque types and constituents may affect the postimplant lumen area, highlighting the important role of lesion preparation to optimize BVS implantation (Fig. 23). In addition, a perfect matching in size between the scaffold and the target vessel is required owing to the reduced device expandability, because postdilation is limited to balloons nr more than 0.5 mm larger than the BVS diameter. OCT has

---

Fig. 17. Optical coherence tomography (OCT)-guided optimization of stent result after percutaneous coronary intervention for ST-elevation myocardial infarction. (A) Coronary angiography after stent implantation within the proximal right coronary artery. (B) Longitudinal reconstruction demonstrates substantial stent malapposition at the proximal edge, extending 5 mm (two white arrows). (C) Cross-section demonstrates stent landing within correct reference segments. (D) Images demonstrate that stent implantation provided full coverage of the thin-capped fibroatheroma (asterisk). (E) Significant plaque protrusion at the culprit site (asterisk). (F) Cross-section of the proximal stent edge demonstrating substantial malapposition, with malapposed area of 3 mm² (arrowhead). (A') Coronary angiography after optimization guided by OCT. (B') Three-dimensional reconstruction of the stented segment reveals uniform stent cell geometry. (C') No further plaque protrusion is observed after dilation with a noncompliant high-pressure balloon. (D') Resolution of residual malapposition at proximal stent edge. (E') Lumen profile shows good stent expansion and acceptable stent minimal luminal area = 7.10 mm²; at distal edge.

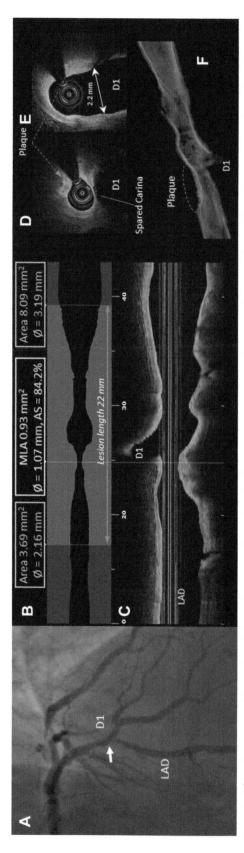

Fig. 18. Bifurcation lesion with sparing of the carina from atherosclerotic disease. (A) Coronary angiography demonstrating a bifurcation lesion involving the left anterior descending (LAD) artery and the first diagonal branch (arrow). (B–E) Baseline optical coherence tomography (OCT) pullback of the LAD. (B, C) Lumen profile and OCT longitudinal view to assess the severity and extension of atherosclerotic involvement. (D, E) OCT cross-sections at the level of bifurcation confirm that the ostium of the first diagonal and the carina are spared from pathology, that the atheroma location is opposite to the takeoff of the first diagonal, and there is no spiky carina that may jeopardize the diagonal during stent placement within the main vessel. (F) Three-dimensional OCT reconstruction provides a 360°panoramic view of the vessel bifurcation segment. Φ, mean diameter; AS, area stenosis; MLA, minimal lumen area.

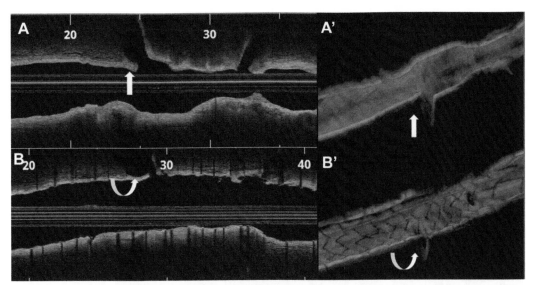

Fig. 19. Carina shift as a mechanism for side-branch compromise after main vessel intervention. (A) Longitudinal view of optical coherence tomography (OCT) pullback of a bifurcation lesion demonstrates a spiky, "eyebrow"-shaped carina extending across the ostium of the side branch, which itself is not involved in the lesion (arrow). (A') Three-dimensional reconstruction of the bifurcation carina at baseline (arrow). (B) After stent implantation, OCT illustrates the effect of the upward shift of the carina after provisional stenting of the main branch (curved arrow). (B') Three-dimensional reconstruction after provisional stenting of the main vessel, showing upward carina shift (curved arrow).

been recommended for BVS size selection and optimization, particularly in complex settings, because a substantial scaffold underexpansion cannot be accommodated with overstretch dilation beyond its designed diameter. In highly complex lesions and patient cohorts (eg, moderate to heavy calcified lesions, bifurcations, chronic total occlusions, and ostial involvement), BVS implantation under OCT guidance, with aggressive lesion preparation, correct BVS sizing and high pressure after dilation, obtained a similar lumen area, percent residual stenosis, and rate of malapposition compared with second-generation drug-eluting stents (Fig. 24).[54] These results achieved with OCT guidance are of paramount importance in light of potential early adverse events after BVS implantation. In a large, multicenter registry of BVS in real-world lesions, the cumulative incidence of definite/probable scaffold thrombosis was 1.5% at 30 days and 2.1% at 6 months, with 16 out of 23 cases occurring within 30 days.[55]

Optical Coherence Tomography after Stent Implantation

OCT during PCI may assess the adequacy of lesion preparation and stent deployment with a high grade of accuracy. In addition to its superiority compared with angiography in detecting residual MLA and minimal lumen diameter, OCT identifies a number of potentially adverse intracoronary features that cannot be detected on angiography (Fig. 25).[20] The goal of OCT performed immediately after stent implantation is to evaluate the adequacy of coronary stent deployment, the full coverage of the diseased segment, stent apposition, stent expansion, stent distortions, edge dissections, tissue protrusion, and the adequacy of access to the side branches. Specifically, OCT detects with high resolution residual MLA, residual area stenosis stent expansion, strut apposition, stent edges dissection, tissue prolapse, residual thrombus, stent distortion and foreshortening, and stent fracture. Table 3 summarizes when and how to intervene based on OCT findings post-stent implantation.

Optical Coherence Tomography to Assess Stent Failure and Vascular Response

OCT can be used for assessing long-term results after stenting and for elucidating the mechanisms underlying stent failure, such as uncovered struts, stent malapposition, and neoatherosclerosis (Fig. 26). Different patterns of neointimal hyperplasia can also be characterized by OCT. Gonzalo and colleagues[56] evaluated the morphologic characteristics of in-stent restenosis (ISR) in 24 patients undergoing OCT imaging (drug-eluting stent, 84%; bare metal stent, 16%). The neointimal tissue was classified

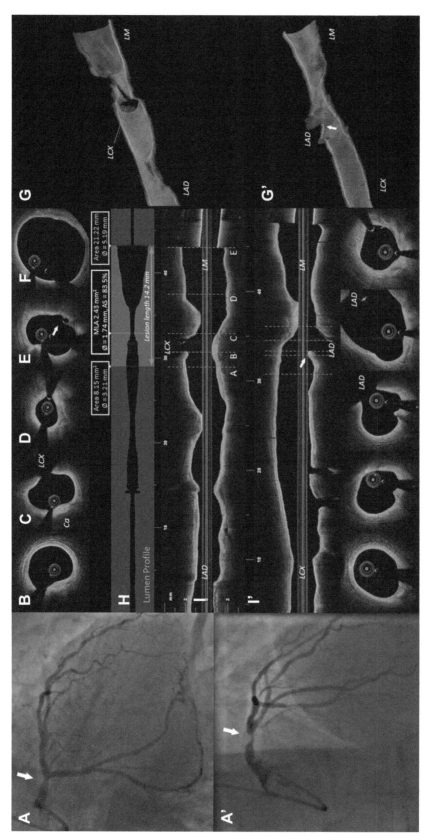

Fig. 20. Optical coherence tomography (OCT)-guided percutaneous coronary intervention to treat the left main bifurcation: vessel assessment. (A, A') Coronary angiography revealed a critical stenosis at the mid-to-distal shaft of the left main coronary artery (arrows in A, A'). OCT pullbacks within left anterior descending (LAD; A) and left circumflex (LCX; A') arteries are shown. (B–F) Cross-sectional images of the OCT pullback within the LAD. (C, D) OCT imaging demonstrates substantial calcified plaque involving the LAD ostium and distal left main carina. (E) Vulnerable plaque with intimal disruption is observed within the left main body (arrow). (H) Lumen profile view of the LAD shows extreme vessel tapering between proximal and distal reference segments (proximal mean diameter 5.19 mm vs distal mean diameter, 3.21 mm). (I) Longitudinal OCT reconstruction of LAD shows distribution of atherosclerotic pahtology. (I') OCT pullback of the LCX displays thick carina protruding into the LM bifurcation (arrow). (G, G') Three-dimensional reconstructions from the perspective of the LAD and LCX, respectively. The protrusion of the carina is well seen in (G'; arrow). Φ, mean diameter; LM, left main; MLA, minimal lumen area.

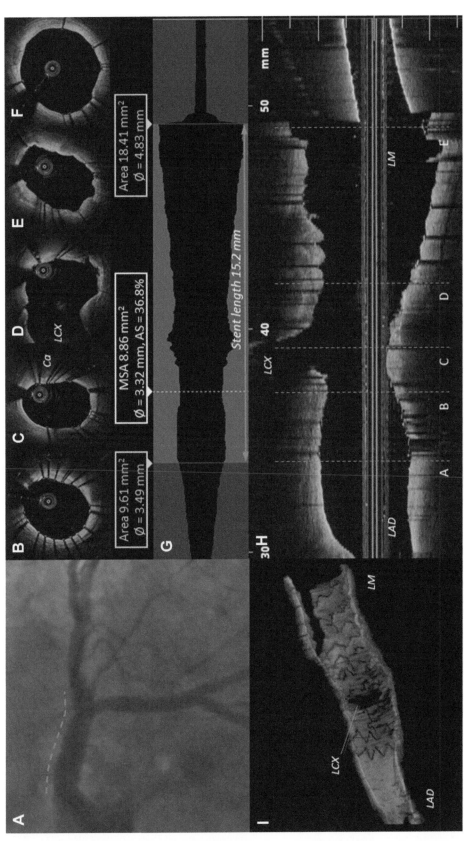

Fig. 21. Optical coherence tomography (OCT)-guided percutaneous coronary intervention to treat left main (LM) bifurcation: Assessment of acute results. (A) Angiogram after drug-eluting stent implantation to treat LM lesion. Dotted line shows the stent position. (B–F) OCT cross-sections of pullback within LAD into LM demonstrate acceptable strut apposition and wide access into the LCX ostium, with no plaque protrusion or dissection. (G) Lumen profile shows acceptable minimal stent area at the ostial LAD (8.9 mm²). (H) Longitudinal reconstruction confirms the absence of edge dissection or malapposition. (I) Three-dimensional reconstruction shows the differential strut cell expansion at within the LM shaft compared with the ostial LAD. Φ, mean diameter; LAD, left anterior descending; LCX, left circumflex; MSA, minimal stent area.

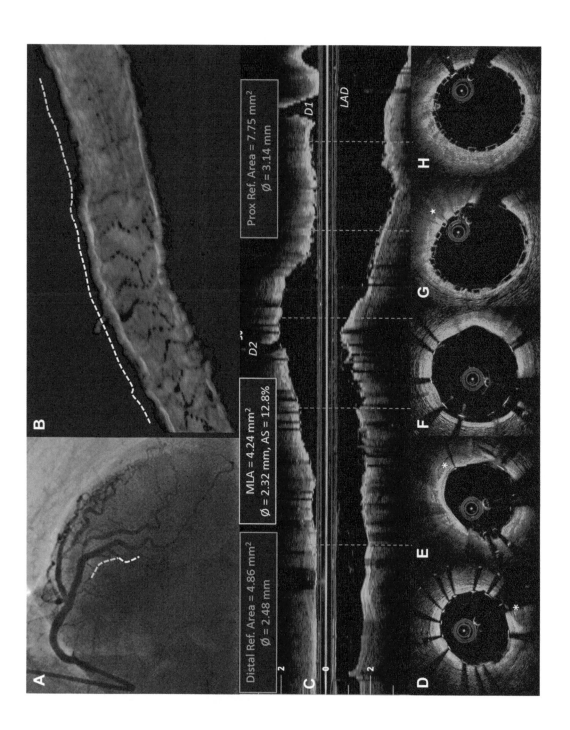

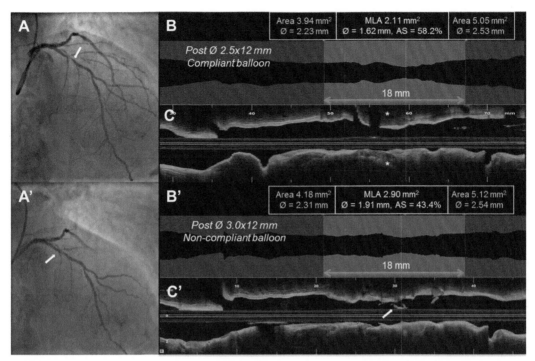

Fig. 23. Optical coherence tomography-guided lesion preparation for BVS implantation. (A) Coronary angiography after lesion dilation with 2.5 mm compliant balloon (arrow). (B) Corresponding automated lumen profile. There is no evidence of substantial plaque modification, and a large residual lesion is still present despite predilatation. (C) Longitudinal view reveals heavy calcification at MLA site (asterisk). (A') Coronary angiography after dilation with a noncompliant 3.0 mm balloon at high pressure (arrow). (B') Automated lumen profile shows improved luminal gain at MLA site. (C') Longitudinal view shows substantial plaque modification, with cracks within calcified lesion (arrow) and no extension of pathology beyond the reference segments. Φ, mean diameter; AS, area stenosis; BVS, bioresorbable vascular scaffold; MLA, minimal lumen area.

according to optical pattern (homogeneous, heterogeneous, or layered), signal backscatter (high or low), the presence or absence of microvessels, lumen shape (regular or irregular), and the presence of intraluminal material. Tissue structure was homogenous in 28%, heterogeneous in 20%, and layered in 52%. The predominant backscatter was high in 72% of cases. This OCT-derived ISR classification has been adopted in subsequent studies and may provide

Fig. 22. BVS and drug-eluting stent (DES) overlap: a hybrid approach for stent selection guided by plaque morphology displayed by optical coherence tomography (OCT). (A) Coronary angiography after DES implantation in distal segment of LAD (white dotted line) overlaps with more proximal BVS (yellow dotted line). (B) Three-dimensional reconstruction displays the 2 stents in overlap. Distal metallic stent (white dotted line) is more visible in the 3-dimensional image than BVS (yellow dotted line). (C) Longitudinal view confirms the good results of both stent implantations. (D, F) OCT cross-sections in the segment treated with the metallic stent displays the calcified lesion beneath stent struts (asterisk). (G, H) OCT cross-sections of the segment treated by BVS displaying the fibrous plaque (star). Φ, mean diameter; AS, area stenosis; BVS, bioresorbable vascular scaffold; LAD, left anterior descending; MLA, minimal lumen area.

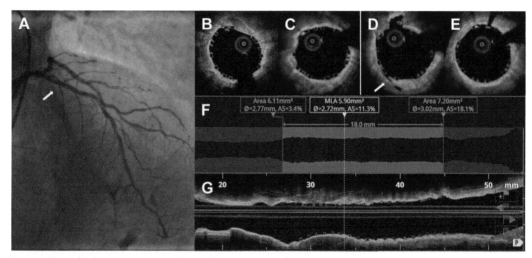

Fig. 24. Optical coherence tomography (OCT) assessment after BVS implantation. (A) Coronary angiography after BVS implantation within proximal LAD (*arrow*). (B, E) OCT cross-sections at the level of reference segments display no dissection or malapposition. (C, D) OCT cross-sections at lesion site display sealing of dissected plaque (*arrow* in D), no malapposition, and excellent acute gain in MLA compared with baseline imaging (not shown). (F) Lumen profile displays excellent acute gain at MLA site (*yellow dashed line*). (G) Longitudinal view confirms the good result of the BVS implantation. Φ, mean diameter; AS, area stenosis; BVS, bioresorbable vascular scaffold; LAD, left anterior descending artery; MLA, minimal lumen area.

insight into guiding the optimal treatment of ISR (eg, the decision on balloon type and stenting technique). Furthermore, OCT is able to provide a detailed assessment of in-stent neoatherosclerosis, which is a common findings in ISR as well as stent thrombosis.[57] Indeed, optical imaging techniques contributed in a substantial way to the identification and characterization of this abnormal neointima growth as a possible causative factor for ST. OCT contributes critically to a reduction in the clinical implications of stent thrombosis with (1) a better mechanistic understanding of the different processes involved (eg, stent underexpansion or malapposition, neoatherosclerosis, strut uncoverage); (2) the identification of surrogate markers anticipating thrombotic risk; and (3) a tailored and more effective approach for the acute treatment of stent thrombosis (Fig. 27).

Recent Innovations and Future Perspectives

Despite a large spectrum of potential advantages, there are still no clear indications for the clinical application of OCT. Currently, there are paucity of data regarding OCT-derived predictors of stent failure, OCT-derived criteria for stent sizing and optimization, and evidence of benefit for OCT-guided PCI on clinical outcomes. No prospective, randomized studies have been performed assessing the role of OCT-guided PCI. At present, interventional cardiologists have to deal with increasingly complex lesions and patient cohorts that require treatment with novel, more technically demanding devices such as BVS, which may require a higher level of accuracy to provide a possibly lower complication rate. This delicate decision-making process can be addressed only by highly detailed information and measurements obtained from rapid and accurate multimodality sources. To this aim, an angiographic–OCT integrated system recently received European Medicines Agency (CE) approval and clearance from the US Food and Drug Administration. This technology departs from the traditional, mobile, cart-based OCT unit. The OPTIS integrated system (St. Jude Medical, St. Paul, MN) offers a direct table control for the entire operation and a fully synchronized co-registration of angiography with OCT (Fig. 28, Video 2). Directly linked visualization of highly accurate vessel morphology with the familiar angiographic lumen profile enables comprehensive integration of OCT into PCI workflow, both before and after intervention.

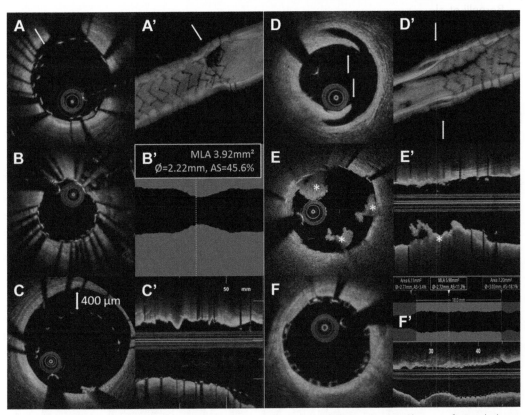

Fig. 25. Optical coherence tomography (OCT) findings after stent implantation. (*A*) Clusters of crowded stent struts that seem to be in overlap at the proximal stent edge (*arrow*); (*A'*) Three-dimensional reconstruction demonstrates stent deformation at proximal edge (*arrow*), explaining the appearance of the stent struts on the cross-sectional image (*A*). (*B*) Stent underexpansion at the level of the calcific lesion. (*B'*) Corresponding lumen profile showing a 45% residual stenosis. (*C*) Large, circumferential stent malapposition (*arrow*). (*C'*) Corresponding longitudinal view showing stent malapposition extending 5 mm longitudinally at the proximal edge. (*D*) Distal edge dissection, involving greater than 2 quadrants and extending deeply into the media (*arrowhead*). (*D'*) Three-dimensional reconstruction showing edge dissection extending 4 mm in length (*arrowhead*). (*E*) New thrombus formation immediately after stent implantation (*asterisk*). (*E'*) Longitudinal view reveals a lipid-rich, thin-capped fibroatheroma at the site of thrombus formation (*asterisk*); (*F*) OCT of a BVS, showing that the polymer boxes are clearly delineated by OCT, without signal attenuation behind struts. (*F'*) Lumen profile and longitudinal reconstruction of the BVS documents full stent expansion and apposition. Φ, mean diameter; AS, area stenosis; BVS, bioresorbable vascular scaffold; MLA, minimal lumen area.

Table 3
Reasonable OCT criteria for intervene during PCI procedures

OCT Findings	Recommendations to Intervene	Recommendations Not to Intervene
Edge dissection	If edge dissection is considered flow limiting	Minor edge dissection that is <180° in <5 frames in OCT
Malapposition	Significant malapposition defined as >200 μm in axial diameter and present in ≥5 consecutive frames on OCT	If malapposition detected is located near a side branch
Thrombus	Presence of thrombus and/or tissue protrusion on OCT causing flow reduction (ie, TIMI <3 and/or obstruction visible by angiography)	Presence of minor thrombus not causing flow reduction
Stent underexpansion	Once OCT shows >30% underexpansion compared with reference distal lumen area and when QCA shows >20% in-stent residual diameter stenosis	In the presence of satisfactory result by QCA, and underexpansion by OCT is <30% area

Abbreviations: OCT, optical coherence tomography; PCI, percutaneous coronary intervention; QCA, quantitative coronary angiogram; TIMI, Thrombolysis In Myocardial Infarction.

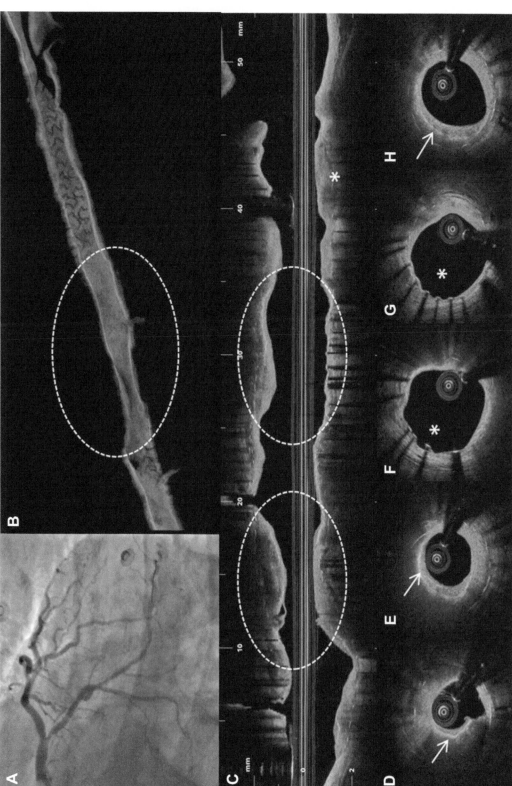

Fig. 26. Very late stent thrombosis owing to drug-eluting stent neoatherosclerosis. (A) Coronary angiography after thrombus aspiration. (B) Three-dimensional reconstruction. (C) Longitudinal view shows multiple in-stent segments that are infiltrated by lipid-laden neointima, that is, neoatherosclerosis (circles). (D–H) Cross-sections substantiate the presence of lipid-rich plaque within the stent, and demonstrate signals of foamy macrophage accumulation (arrows). (F, G) Cross-sections of stented segment showing uncovered stent struts (asterisk).

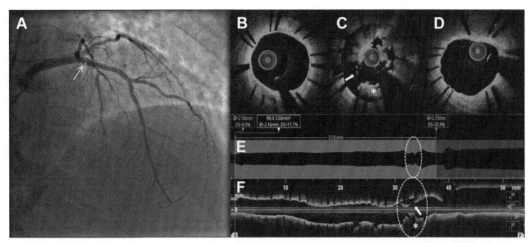

Fig. 27. Drug-eluting stent thrombosis owing to persistent malapposition. (A) Angiography of the left anterior descending after thrombus aspiration shows persistent haziness at the level of an aneurysm located at the stent entrance (arrow). (B–D) Cross-sectional images. (E) Lumen profile. (F) Longitudinal view. (B, D) Optimal healing and coverage of the stented segment at both distal and proximal sites. (C) Cluster of grossly malapposed and uncovered struts (arrow) with large residual thrombus despite thrombus aspiration (asterisk). Automatic lumen profile (E) and longitudinal view (F) show uniform stent expansion, except for the segment at the level of the aneurysm (arrow) and thrombus (asterisk, circle).

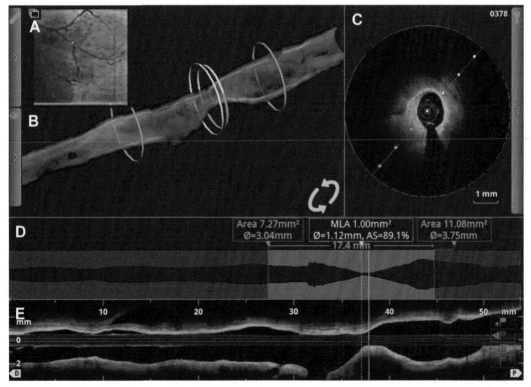

Fig. 28. Co-registration of angiography with optical coherence tomography (OCT). (A) Coronary angiography synchronized with OCT pullback within the left circumflex. Angiography co-registration works by tracking the radiopaque lens marker of the Dragonfly OPTIS or Dragonfly DUO catheter within a cine-angiogram acquired during the OCT pullback. The white hashmark within the left circumflex represents the location of the OCT imaging element and corresponds with the concurrent OCT image. (B) Real-time 3-dimensional reconstruction provides a 360-degree panoramic view of the vessel. The yellow-and-blue arc corresponds with the white hashmark on the angiogram, the yellow-and-blue line on the longitudinal reconstruction, and the currently displayed cross-sectional image. (C) Lumen profile. (D) Longitudinal reconstruction displays the extension of the disease. (E) Cross-sectional image providing information regarding lesion morphology at the site of the white hashmark on angiography.

SUMMARY

OCT is a unique intracoronary imaging technique that provides high-resolution, easy-to-interpret images that can be translated into clinical practice for the planning and mapping of complex PCI procedures. The precise morphologic information obtained across long segments of the coronary vessels, combined with automatic measurements and enhanced software capabilities (eg, real-time 3D reconstruction and co-registration with angiography), makes OCT more than an additional and promising intravascular tool for PCI guidance. The new integrated co-registration system that synchronizes OCT with coronary angiography may set a new standard for routine adoption of imaging guidance and stent optimization in PCI. Whether OCT-guided PCI will lead to superior clinical outcomes compared with angiography alone in the contemporary era of new-generation drug-eluting stent and BVS, as well as potent adjunct pharmacology, remains to be proven with large, prospective, randomized clinical trials. However, OCT criteria for stent optimization, based on preprocedural and postprocedural assessments, have been tested in prospective registries.

SUPPLEMENTARY DATA

Supplementary data related to this article can be found online at http://dx.doi.org/10.1016/j.iccl.2015.02.008.

REFERENCES

1. Garrone P, Biondi-Zoccai G, Salvetti I, et al. Quantitative coronary angiography in the current era: principles and applications. J Interv Cardiol 2009; 22:527–36.
2. Witzenbichler B, Maehara A, Weisz G, et al. Relationship between intravascular ultrasound guidance and clinical outcomes after drug-eluting stents: the assessment of dual antiplatelet therapy with drug-eluting stents (ADAPT-DES) study. Circulation 2014;28(129):463–70.
3. Prati F, Guagliumi G, Mintz GS, et al. Expert review document part 2: methodology, terminology and clinical applications of optical coherence tomography for the assessment of interventional procedures. Eur Heart J 2012;33:2513–20.
4. Gutiérrez H, Arnold R, Gimeno F, et al. Optical coherence tomography. Initial experience in patients undergoing percutaneous coronary intervention. Rev Esp Cardiol 2008;61:976–9.
5. MacNeill BD, Lowe HC, Takano M, et al. Intravascular modalities for detection of vulnerable plaque: current status. Arterioscler Thromb Vasc Biol 2003; 23:1333–42.
6. Jang IK, Bouma BE, Kang DH, et al. Visualization of coronary atherosclerotic plaques in patients using optical coherence tomography: comparison with intravascular ultrasound. J Am Coll Cardiol 2002; 39:604–9.
7. Tearney GJ, Yabushita H, Houser SL, et al. Quantification of macrophage content in atherosclerotic plaques by optical coherence tomography. Circulation 2003;107:113–9.
8. Bouma BE, Tearney GJ, Yabushita H, et al. Evaluation of intracoronary stenting by intravascular optical coherence tomography. Heart 2003;89:317–21.
9. Barlis P, Schmitt JM. Current and future developments in intracoronary optical coherence tomography imaging. EuroIntervention 2009;4:529–33.
10. Radu MD, Raber L, Heo J, et al. Natural history of optical coherence tomography-detected non-flow-limiting edge dissections following drug-eluting stent implantation. EuroIntervention 2014; 9(9):1085–94.
11. Windecker S, Kolh P, Alfonso F, et al. 2014 ESC/EACTS Guidelines on myocardial revascularization: The Task Force on Myocardial Revascularization of the European Society of Cardiology (ESC) and the European Association for Cardio-Thoracic Surgery (EACTS) Developed with the special contribution of the European Association of Percutaneous Cardiovascular Interventions (EAPCI). Eur Heart J 2014;1(35):2541–619.
12. Montalescot G, Sechtem U, Achenbach S, et al. 2013 ESC guidelines on the management of stable coronary artery disease: the Task Force on the management of stable coronary artery disease of the European Society of Cardiology. Eur Heart J 2013;34:2949–3003.
13. Lotfi A, Jeremias A, Fearon WF, et al. Expert consensus statement on the use of fractional flow reserve, intravascular ultrasound, and optical coherence tomography: a consensus statement of the Society of Cardiovascular Angiography and Interventions. Catheter Cardiovasc Interv 2014;1(83): 509–18.
14. Imola F, Mallus MT, Ramazzotti V, et al. Safety and feasibility of frequency domain optical coherence tomography to guide decision making in percutaneous coronary intervention. EuroIntervention 2010;6:575–81.
15. Stefano GT, Bezerra HG, Mehanna E, et al. Unrestricted utilization of frequency domain optical coherence tomography in coronary interventions. Int J Cardiovasc Imaging 2013;29(4):741–52.
16. Viceconte N, Chan PH, Barrero EA, et al. Frequency domain optical coherence tomography for guidance of coronary stenting. Int J Cardiol 2013; 1(166):722–8.

17. Prati F, Di Vito L, Biondi-Zoccai G, et al. Angiography alone versus angiography plus optical coherence tomography to guide decision-making during percutaneous coronary intervention: the centro per la lotta contro l'infarto-optimisation of percutaneous coronary intervention (CLI-OPCI) study. EuroIntervention 2012;8:823–9.

18. Räber L, Radu MD. Optimising cardiovascular outcomes using optical coherence tomography-guided percutaneous coronary interventions. EuroIntervention 2012;22(8):765–71.

19. Fedele S, Biondi-Zoccai G, Kwiatkowski P, et al. Reproducibility of coronary optical coherence tomography for lumen and length measurements in humans (The CLI-VAR [Centro per la Lotta contro l'Infarto-VARiability] study). Am J Cardiol 2012; 15(110):1106–12.

20. Gonzalo N, Garcia-Garcia HM, Serruys PW, et al. Reproducibility of quantitative optical coherence tomography for stent analysis. EuroIntervention 2009;5:224–32.

21. Kubo T, Akasaka T, Shite J, et al. OCT compared with IVUS in a coronary lesion assessment: the OPUS-CLASS study. JACC Cardiovasc Imaging 2013;6:1095–104.

22. Bezerra HG, Attizzani GF, Sirbu V, et al. Optical coherence tomography versus intravascular ultrasound to evaluate coronary artery disease and percutaneous coronary intervention. JACC Cardiovasc Interv 2013;6:228–36.

23. Yabushita H, Bouma BE, Houser SL, et al. Characterization of human atherosclerosis by optical coherence tomography. Circulation 2002;106:1640–5.

24. Kume T, Akasaka T, Kawamoto T, et al. Assessment of coronary intima-media thickness by optical coherence tomography: comparison with intravascular ultrasound. Circ J 2005;69:903–7.

25. Cilingiroglu M, Oh JH, Sugunan B, et al. Detection of vulnerable plaque in a murine model of atherosclerosis with optical coherence tomography. Catheter Cardiovasc Interv 2006;67:915–23.

26. Kume T, Akasaka T, Kawamoto T, et al. Measurement of the thickness of the fibrous cap by optical coherence tomography. Am Heart J 2006;152(755): e751–4.

27. MacNeill BD, Jang IK, Bouma BE, et al. Focal and multi-focal plaque macrophage distributions in patients with acute and stable presentations of coronary artery disease. J Am Coll Cardiol 2004;44:972–9.

28. Ishibashi K, Kitabata H, Akasaka T. Intracoronary optical coherence tomography assessment of spontaneous coronary artery dissection. Heart 2009;95:818.

29. Bernelli C, Komukai K, Sirbu V, et al. Coronary artery disease in systemic sclerosis not clinically apparent: findings from optical coherence tomography. Eur Heart J 2014;35:764.

30. Stefano GT, Bezerra HG, Attizzani G, et al. Utilization of frequency domain optical coherence tomography and fractional flow reserve to assess intermediate coronary artery stenoses: conciliating anatomic and physiologic information. Int J Cardiovasc Imaging 2011;27:299–308.

31. Porto I, Di Vito L, Burzotta F, et al. Predictors of periprocedural (type IVa) myocardial infarction, as assessed by frequency-domain optical coherence tomography. Circ Cardiovasc Interv 2012;5:89–96. S1–6.

32. Joner M, Finn AV, Farb A, et al. Pathology of drug-eluting stents in humans: delayed healing and late thrombotic risk. J Am Coll Cardiol 2006;48:193–202.

33. Tanaka A, Imanishi T, Kitabata H, et al. Lipid-rich plaque and myocardial perfusion after successful stenting in patients with non-ST segment elevation acute coronary syndrome: an optical coherence tomography study. Eur Heart J 2009;30: 1348–55.

34. Tearney GJ, Regar E, Akasaka T, et al. Consensus standards for acquisition, measurement, and reporting of intravascular optical coherence tomography studies: a report from the international working group for intravascular optical coherence tomography standardization and validation. J Am Coll Cardiol 2012;59:1058–72.

35. Gonzalo N, Serruys PW, Okamura T, et al. Relation between plaque type and dissections at the edges after stent implantation: an optical coherence tomography study. Int J Cardiol 2011;150:151–5.

36. Chamié D, Bezerra HG, Attizzani GF, et al. Incidence, predictors, morphological characteristics, and clinical outcomes of stent edge dissections detected by optical coherence tomography. JACC Cardiovasc Interv 2013;6:800–13.

37. Kume T, Okura H, Kawamoto T, et al. Assessment of the coronary calcification by optical coherence tomography. EuroIntervention 2011;6:768–72.

38. Martín-Yuste V, Barros A, Leta R, et al. Factors determining success in percutaneous revascularization of chronic total coronary occlusion: multidetector computed tomography analysis. Rev Esp Cardiol 2012;65:334–40.

39. Tenaglia AN, Buller CE, Kisslo KB, et al. Intracoronary ultrasound predictors of adverse outcomes after coronary artery interventions. J Am Coll Cardiol 1992;20:1385–94.

40. Kubo T, Imanishi T, Takarada S, et al. Assessment of culprit lesion morphology in acute myocardial infarction: ability of optical coherence tomography compared with intravascular ultrasound and coronary angioscopy. J Am Coll Cardiol 2007;50: 933–9.

41. Kato K, Yonetsu T, Kim SJ, et al. Non culprit plaques in patients with acute coronary syndromes

have more vulnerable features compared with those with non-acute coronary syndromes: A 3-vessel optical coherence tomography study. Circ Cardiovasc Imaging 2012;5:433–40.

42. Jia H, Abtahian F, Aguirre AD, et al. In vivo diagnosis of plaque erosion and calcified nodule in patients with acute coronary syndrome by intravascular optical coherence tomography. J Am Coll Cardiol 2013;62:1748–58.

43. Onuma Y, Thuesen L, van Geuns RJ, et al, TROFI Investigators. Randomized study to assess the effect of thrombus aspiration on flow area in patients with ST-elevation myocardial infarction: an optical frequency domain imaging study–TROFI trial. Eur Heart J 2013;34:1050–60.

44. Magro M, Regar E, Gutiérrez-Chico JL, et al. Residual atherothrombotic material after stenting in acute myocardial infarction-an optical coherence tomographic evaluation. Int J Cardiol 2013;167:656–63.

45. Nakazawa G, Finn AV, Joner M, et al. Delayed arterial healing and increased late stent thrombosis at culprit sites after drug-eluting stent placement for acute myocardial infarction patients: an autopsy study. Circulation 2008;118:1138–45.

46. Gonzalo N, Barlis P, Serruys PW, et al. Incomplete stent apposition and delayed tissue coverage are more frequent in drug-eluting stents implanted during primary percutaneous coronary intervention for ST-segment elevation myocardial infarction than in drug-eluting stents implanted for stable/unstable angina: insights from optical coherence tomography. JACC Cardiovasc Interv 2009;2:445–52.

47. Nakazawa G, Yazdani SK, Finn AV, et al. Pathological findings at bifurcation lesions: the impact of flow distribution on atherosclerosis and arterial healing after stent implantation. J Am Coll Cardiol 2010;55:1679–87.

48. Medina A, Martín P, Suárez de Lezo J, et al. Vulnerable carina anatomy and ostial lesions in the left anterior descending coronary artery after floating-stent treatment. Rev Esp Cardiol 2009;62:1240–9.

49. Di Mario C, Iakovou I, van der Giessen WJ, et al. Optical coherence tomography for guidance in bifurcation lesion treatment. EuroIntervention 2010;6(Suppl J):J99–106.

50. Farooq V, Serruys PW, Heo JH, et al. New insights into the coronary artery bifurcation hypothesis-generating concepts utilizing 3-dimensional optical frequency domain imaging. JACC Cardiovasc Interv 2011;4:921–31.

51. Karanasos A, Tu S, van der Heide E, et al. Carina shift as a mechanism for side-branch compromise following main vessel intervention: insights from three-dimensional optical coherence tomography. Cardiovasc Diagn Ther 2012;2:173–7.

52. Hariki H, Shinke T, Otake H, et al. Potential benefit of final kissing balloon inflation after single stenting for the treatment of bifurcation lesions-insights from optical coherence tomography observations. Circ J 2013;77:1193–201.

53. Fujino Y, Bezerra HG, Attizzani GF, et al. Frequency-domain optical coherence tomography assessment of unprotected left main coronary artery disease-a comparison with intravascular ultrasound. Catheter Cardiovasc Interv 2013;82:E173–83.

54. Mattesini A, Secco GG, Dall'Ara G, et al. ABSORB biodegradable stents versus second-generation metal stents: a comparison study of 100 complex lesions treated under OCT guidance. JACC Cardiovasc Interv 2014;7:741–50.

55. Capodanno D, Gori T, Nef H, et al. Percutaneous coronary intervention with everolimus-eluting bioresorbable vascular scaffolds in routine clinical practice: early and midterm outcomes from the European multicentre GHOST-EU registry. EuroIntervention 2015;10(11):1144–53.

56. Gonzalo N, Serruys PW, Okamura T, et al. Optical coherence tomography patterns of stent restenosis. Am Heart J 2009;158:284–93.

57. Komukai K, Bernelli C, Sirbu V, et al. Stent Failure due to Simultaneous Aggressive Neoatherosclerosis of First and Current Generation Drug Eluting Stents. Eurointervention, in press.

Assessment and Quantitation of Stent Results by Intracoronary Optical Coherence Tomography

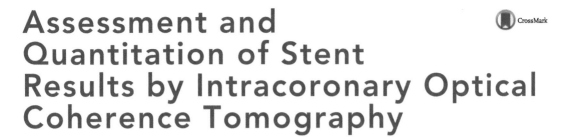

Akiko Maehara, MD[a,b,*], Mitsuaki Matsumura, BS[b],
Gary S. Mintz, MD[b]

KEYWORDS

• OCT • Stent • Dissection • Malapposition

KEY POINTS

- Important characteristics that should be evaluated as part of a formal quantitative optical coherence tomography (OCT) analysis poststenting include stent expansion and stent malapposition; qualitative analysis includes the evaluation of tissue protrusion, thrombus evaluation, and stent edge dissection.
- Stent expansion is expressed as the absolute minimum stent area (MSA) ratio, which compares the MSA with the reference lumen area or the mean stent area determined by volumetric analysis.
- Stent strut malapposition is present when the distance from the center of the blooming artifact of the stent to the surface of the lumen or adjacent plaque is greater than the sum of the known stent thickness and polymer thickness. Malappositon may also be reported as percent of total struts that are malapposed within the entire stent, or the percent malapposition area.
- Tissue protrusion can be described as percent tissue protrusion area, defined as the maximum tissue protrusion area divided by the stent area, and the residual effective lumen area, which is defined as the minimum lumen area within the region of tissue protrusion.
- Other OCT poststent qualitative evaluations include tissue protrusion (either plaque or thrombus) through the stent strut, semiquantitative thrombus evaluation, and stent edge dissection.
- Thrombus is defined as intraluminal tissue greater than 0.25 mm in diameter, with high backscatter and high attenuation (red-cell–rich thrombus), less backscatter with low attenuation (platelet-rich thrombus), or a mixture of both.
- Stent edge dissection is commonly observed on OCT; the severity of a dissection should be assessed by evaluation of dissection depth (intimal or into the medial); the angle of dissection flap; the residual effective lumen area inside of the dissection; and longitudinal length of the dissection.

Dr A. Maehara has received research funding from Boston Scientific, is a consultant for Boston Scientific and ACIST, and has received speaker fees from St. Jude Medical. Dr G.S. Mintz has received research funding from and is a consultant for Boston Scientific. Dr M. Matsumura has nothing to disclose.
[a] Department of Medicine, Columbia University Medical Center, 161 Fort Washington Avenue, New York, NY 10032, USA; [b] Clinical Trials Center, Cardiovascular Research Foundation, 111 East 59th Street, 12th Floor, New York, NY 10022, USA
* Corresponding author. 111 East 59th Street, 12th Floor, New York, NY 10022.
E-mail address: amaehara@crf.org

Intervent Cardiol Clin 4 (2015) 285–294
http://dx.doi.org/10.1016/j.iccl.2015.02.003

INTRODUCTION

Because most imaging data has been based on intravascular ultrasound (IVUS) studies,[1–8] the difference between optical coherence tomography (OCT) and IVUS should be recognized to better understand the results of OCT image analysis. The main difference between OCT and IVUS is a ten-fold better resolution with worse penetration.[9–11] In studies in which OCT and IVUS were compared in vivo, the mean differences in lumen area varied from 0.19 mm^2 to 1.15 mm^2; lumen area was consistently larger with IVUS than OCT, especially in smaller lumens and in nonstented segments.[12–16]

In addition to these differences in quantitative measurements, the incidence of certain qualitative poststent findings was more frequent with OCT. Kubo and colleagues[16] evaluated 100 patients with both OCT and IVUS and reported that the prevalence of tissue protrusion (95% vs 18%; P<.001), incomplete stent apposition (39% vs 14%; P<.001), stent edge dissection (13% vs 0%; P = .0013), and intrastent thrombus (13% vs 0%; P = .013) were greater by OCT compared with IVUS.[15–21]

Another important characteristic of OCT is that interobserver and intraobserver variability is better compared with that of IVUS.[16,22,23] The deviation between independent measurements of lumen area by IVUS was approximately twice as high compared with measurements by OCT.[16] Because the clearance of blood by flushing with contrast or dextran is required for OCT imaging, the border between the lumen and vessel structure is clearer than with IVUS, resulting in not only less variability of diagnosis, but also acceptable automatic contouring of the

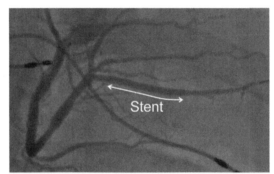

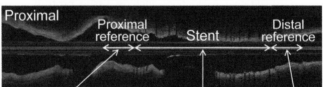

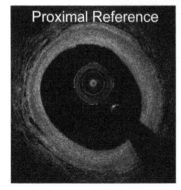
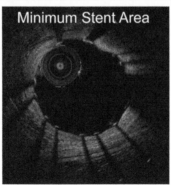
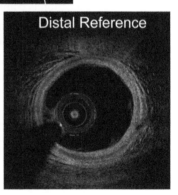

Fig. 1. Poststent OCT image with corresponding coronary angiography. After the entire stent segment is reviewed, the key slices having the minimum stent area, minimum lumen area, and proximal and distal most normal-looking slice are chosen and analyzed. The most normal-looking slices are defined as the slices having the largest lumen area within 5 mm of the stent edge but before a significant side branch. In this case, the minimum stent area slice is located in the middle of the stent.

lumen border in most cases. However, a major drawback of OCT is less image penetration, and one often cannot evaluate vessel size according to media-to-media diameter; nor can one quantitate plaque burden, which has been shown to be an important predictor of future events.[24]

STENT EXPANSION

Fig. 1 shows an example of a poststent OCT image with corresponding coronary angiography. After reviewing the entire stent segment, one compares the visualized stent length with the reported stent length. If the difference between the lengths is less than 10%, one may consider the automatic pullback reliable and proceed with volumetric analysis. Stent length measurements based on known pullback speed and frame rates have been reported to be very accurate, with a mean difference between actual stent length and OCT-measured stent length of 0.15 ± 0.68 mm (less than 1% of length) in 77 lesions using a single stent as a reference (19.8 $\pm$ 5.6 mm).[23] The stent segment is defined as the segment between the first and last frames in which at least 70% of stent struts are visualized in a single cross-sectional image. The

5-mm segments beyond the stent edges before a significant side branch (defined as a side branch >1.5 mm in diameter) are considered proximal and distal references. Volumetric analysis includes lumen and stent contours every 1 mm, and lumen or stent volume is calculated using the Simpson rule. One commonly reports volumetric data as a mean value defined by total stent or lumen volume divided by the analyzed stent length to normalize for differences in stent length. A slice having the smallest lumen and/or stent area is chosen and reported as a key measurement that relates to outcomes. Sawada and colleagues[25] evaluated the accuracy of stent measurement by OCT using stents implanted into a rubber arterial phantom model and confirmed that the stent surface should be measured at the center of stent blooming artifact. Based on this evidence, we analyze stent area by connecting to the center of each blooming artifact. Fig. 2 shows the contouring of stent area.

Stent expansion is calculated as minimum stent area (MSA) divided by the average reference lumen area multiplied by 100. The reference lumen area is determined from the most normal-looking slice within the reference segment, which is defined as the slice having

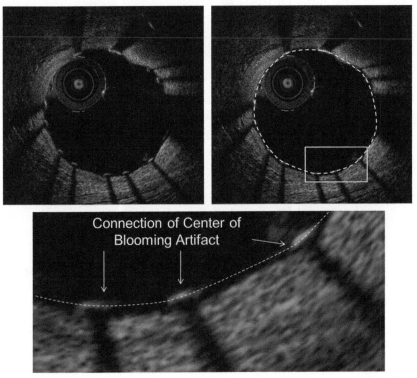

Fig. 2. Stent contouring. A stent is contoured by connecting the center of the blooming artifact of each stent strut (dotted line).

the largest lumen area, because the external elastic membrane (EEM) is not always visible by OCT and plaque burden cannot be evaluated even in the reference segments. **Fig. 3** shows the measurements of MSA and lumen areas at the proximal and distal reference (most normal-looking) slices.

IVUS studies have demonstrated that the strongest procedural predictor of stent thrombosis and restenosis is the MSA achieved after percutaneous coronary intervention (PCI).[1–4] By achieving greater stent luminal dimensions, IVUS guidance has been associated with improved outcomes.[5–8] Based on IVUS studies, the definition of optimal stent expansion according to OCT was proposed to be MSA greater than or equal to 90% of distal reference lumen area or MSA greater than or equal to 90% of the average of reference lumen area.[26,27] To choose the appropriate size of balloon or stent, the lumen diameter and/or EEM diameter of the

reference segment may be used. Habara and colleagues[27] conducted a randomized study of 70 patients that compared OCT- with IVUS-guided stenting in de novo coronary artery lesions. In this study, good EEM visibility (defined as ≥270 degrees of EEM circumference visible) before PCI was present in only 63% of cases, and stent size was chosen based on angiography for the 37% of the cases with poor EEM visibility, resulting in a smaller final MSA with OCT guidance compared with IVUS guidance (5.7 ± 2.1 vs 6.9 ± 2.4 mm²; $P = .03$, comparing MSAs measured in both groups by OCT). Recently, Kubo and colleagues[28] showed good estimation of unidentified circular arc of EEM area (vessel area) based on the curvature of visible EEM segment, and therefore this may be a promising approach to EEM identification and subsequent device sizing. The use of OCT measurements to choose an appropriate balloon/stent size requires further research.

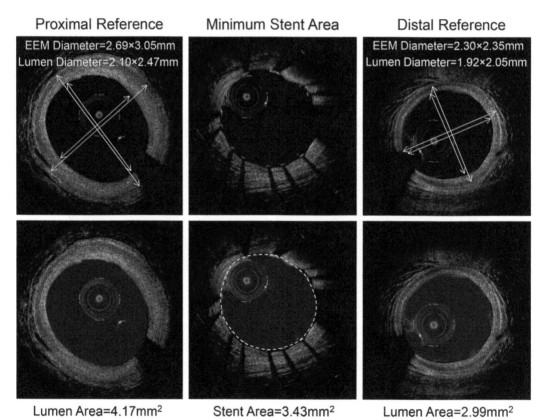

Proximal Reference   **Minimum Stent Area**   **Distal Reference**

EEM Diameter=2.69×3.05mm
Lumen Diameter=2.10×2.47mm

EEM Diameter=2.30×2.35mm
Lumen Diameter=1.92×2.05mm

Lumen Area=4.17mm²   Stent Area=3.43mm²   Lumen Area=2.99mm²

Fig. 3. Measurement of MSA (*dotted line*) and proximal and distal reference sites. MSA measures 3.43 mm², and the proximal and distal lumen areas at the most normal-looking slice measure 4.17 and 2.99 mm², respectively, for an average reference lumen area of (4.17 + 2.99)/2 = 3.58 mm². Therefore, stent expansion for this stent is calculated as MSA/(average of reference lumen area) × 100 = 3.43/3.58 × 100 = 95.8%. Minimum and maximum lumen diameters (*white arrows*) and EEM diameters (*yellow arrows*). In this case at proximal and distal references the media is visible, and lumen and EEM diameters can be analyzed as shown (proximal and distal mean diameter of lumen/EEM = 2.29/2.87 and 1.99/2.33 mm, respectively).

STENT MALAPPOSITION

The actual thickness of the stent (sum of strut thickness and polymer thickness) is not visualized by OCT because of signal attenuation behind the stent struts.[9–11] Therefore, malapposition can be determined to be present when the distance from the center of blooming artifact of the stent strut to the surface of the adjacent plaque is greater than the sum of the known strut thickness and polymer thickness. Typically, malappositon is reported as the percent of total strut that is malapposed within the entire stent.[19–21] In addition, to quantify the severity of malapposition, percent maximum malapposition area is defined as the maximum malapposition area divided by the lumen area at the same slice, and the total malapposed length is measured. Fig. 4 shows an example of stent strut malapposition analysis.

Because of its higher resolution, OCT can identify acute stent malapposition much more frequently compared with IVUS[16–21]; however, numerous IVUS and OCT studies have confirmed that acute stent malapposition, when it does not accompany stent underexpansion, does not correlate with early stent thrombosis or subsequent restenosis.[29,30] Im and colleagues[19] evaluated 351 patients treated by drug-eluting stents with baseline and 6-month follow-up OCT. Acute stent malapposition was observed in 62% of lesions (percentage of acute malapposed struts, 5.2% ± 6.2%), and half of acute malapposition was located at the stent edge. At follow-up, one-third of acute malapposition persisted, and the rate of persistence was related to the magnitude of the acute malapposition. Late-acquired malapposition (ie, only visible at follow-up) was found in 15% of lesions, mainly

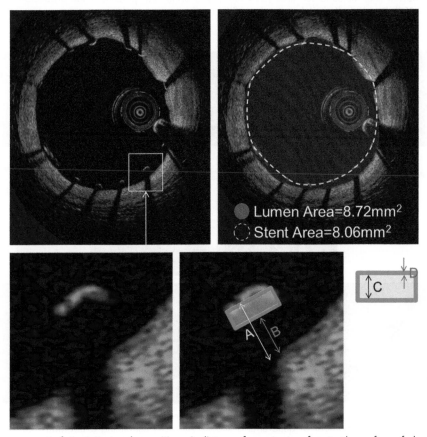

Lumen Area=8.72mm²
Stent Area=8.06mm²

Fig. 4. Measurement of stent strut malapposition. *A*, distance from stent surface to the surface of plaque; *B*, malapposition distance; *C*, strut thickness; *D*, polymer thickness. Because of attenuation behind stent struts, the actual thickness of the stent (sum of strut thickness and polymer thickness) is not visualized by optical coherence tomography. Therefore, *A* is measured; *B* is calculated by subtracting *C* + *D* from *A*; and if *B* >0, the strut is diagnosed as malapposed. Percent maximum malapposed area, defined as maximum malapposed area ([lumen area – stent area]/lumen area × 100), and total malapposed length (the length having consecutive visible malapposed struts) can be determined. In this case, malapposition area (0.66 mm²) was calculated as lumen area (8.72 mm², shown in *gray*) subtracted from the stent area (8.06 mm² shown in the *dotted area*).

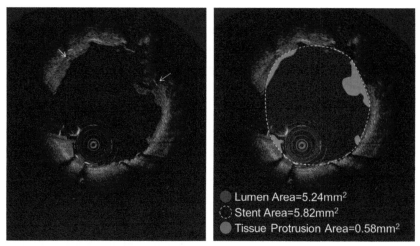

Fig. 5. Tissue protrusion. Tissue protrusion is defined as a tissue (either plaque or thrombus) through the stent strut (*arrows*). To evaluate the significance of tissue protrusion, percent tissue protrusion area (tissue protrusion area/ stent area × 100) is calculated. Tissue protrusion area (0.58 mm^2, *green area*) is calculated as stent area (5.82 mm^2, *dotted line*) minus lumen area (5.24 mm^2, *gray area*), and percent tissue protrusion area is 10.0% (0.58/5.82 × 100). Residual effective lumen area is 5.24 mm^2.

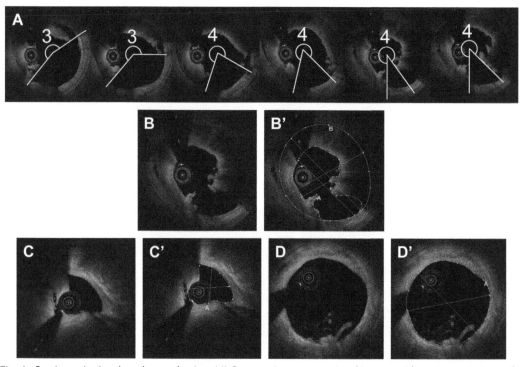

Fig. 6. Semiquantitative thrombus evaluation. (A) Consecutive cross-sectional images with semiquantitaive evaluation of thrombus by the number of quadrants is shown. All slices containing a thrombus are evaluated and summed. For example, in this case the total score is 22 (3+3+4+4+4+4 = 22). (B) The slice containing maximum thrombus area is within A. If the outline of the thrombus is visible, the slice with maximum thrombus is chosen and analyzed by subtracting the lumen area from the area of the outline of the thrombus (B'). If the outline of a thrombus is not visible (as it is in B), the minimum lumen area within the thrombus (C) is chosen, and the maximum thrombus area is calculated by subtracting the minimum lumen area (C') from the visible lumen area (D', not including thrombus) at the closest adjacent reference site (D). (*Adapted from* Parodi G, Valenti R, Migliorini A, et al. Comparison of manual thrombus aspiration with rheolytic thrombectomy in acute myocardial infarction. Circ Cardiovasc Interv 2013;6:224–30; with permission.)

in the body of the stent, was related to baseline tissue and/or thrombus protrusion through the stent struts, but was not related to subsequent clinical outcomes at 2.4 ± 0.9 years of follow-up. This observation is consistent with prior IVUS reports.[29,30]

TISSUE PROTRUSION

Tissue protrusion is diagnosed whenever tissue is seen within the stent struts. The protruded material can be either thrombus or plaque. To evaluate the significance of tissue protrusion, percent tissue protrusion area is defined as maximum tissue protrusion area divided by the stent area, and residual effective lumen area is defined as the minimum lumen area within the tissue protrusion (Fig. 5).

IVUS studies have reported that as long as the residual lumen area is large enough (>5 mm²),

tissue protrusion is not related to stent thrombosis, and resolves at follow-up.[4,31] By OCT, Sugiyama and colleagues[32] evaluated 178 patients (87% with stable angina) treated by drug-eluting stents with normal pre-PCI creatine kinase-MB. The independent morphologic predictors of tissue protrusion included right coronary artery location, lesion length, and thin-cap fibroatheroma. Although lesions with post-PCI creatine kinase-MB elevation more than the upper reference limit showed larger amounts of tissue protrusion, there was no difference in cardiac events between the patients with versus without tissue protrusion. Onuma and colleagues[33] evaluated the efficacy of thrombectomy before stenting in 141 patients with ST elevation myocardial infarction less than 12 hours from onset who were randomized to primary PCI with or without thrombectomy. The primary end point, defined as minimum flow area (stent area

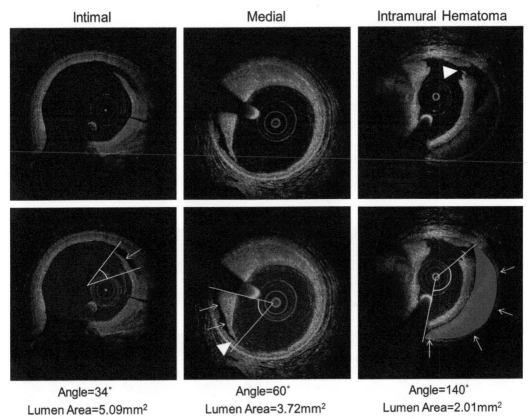

Intimal	Medial	Intramural Hematoma
Angle=34°	Angle=60°	Angle=140°
Lumen Area=5.09mm²	Lumen Area=3.72mm²	Lumen Area=2.01mm²

Fig. 7. Classification of stent edge dissection. Based on the depth of dissection, stent edge dissection is categorized as intimal or medial. *Left*, intimal dissection is observed in the reference segment. The angle of the flap (*arrow*) is 34 degrees, and the effective lumen area (*gray area*) within the dissection flap is 5.09 mm². *Middle*, medial dissection has reached the medial plane, identified by comparing the adjacent circumference medial border (*white triangle*). The angle of dissection flap (*arrows*) is measured as 60 degrees, and the effective lumen area is 3.72 mm². *Right*, intramural hematoma. The entry site of the hematoma (*white triangle*) has reached the media. A hematoma can be observed within the media (*green area*) and has pushed the lumen inward. The angle of dissection (*arrows*) is measured as 140 degrees, and the effective lumen area is 2.01 mm².

minus tissue protrusion area within the stent), did not differ between the two groups, and total tissue protrusion volume was also similar (with vs without thrombectomy; 5.27 ± 4.20 vs 5.55 ± 5.65 mm³; P = .75).

THROMBUS EVALUATION

Evaluation of thrombus by OCT has been reported as accurate, and red-cell–rich thrombus can be differentiated compared with platelet-rich thrombus.[9–11,34,35] Thrombus is defined as intraluminal tissue greater than 0.25 mm in diameter and either high backscattering with high attenuation (red-cell–rich thrombus), less backscattering with homogeneous low attenuation (platelet-rich thrombus), or a mixture of both. After reviewing the entire lesion segment, the segment containing any amount of thrombus is identified. Each slice is subdivided into four quadrants, the presence or absence of thrombus tabulated per quadrant, and the total number of quadrants containing thrombus is summed. In addition, the maximum thrombus area is calculated by tracing the outline of the thrombus if the outline is visible, or subtracting the minimum lumen area within the thrombus from the adjacent reference lumen area not having thrombus if the outline of thrombus is not visible (Fig. 6). Using this method, we have reported that rheolytic thrombectomy shows less residual thrombus burden compared with manual thrombus aspiration.[35]

STENT EDGE DISSECTION

Stent edge dissection by OCT can be categorized as intimal or medial. The depth of dissection is within the intima for intimal dissection, and the dissection reaches to the media or demonstrates an intramural hematoma in the case of medial dissection. Defining the depth of the dissection requires that the media adjacent to the dissection be recognized. An intramural hematoma is one type of medial dissection that extends within the media longitudinally, typically without a re-entry

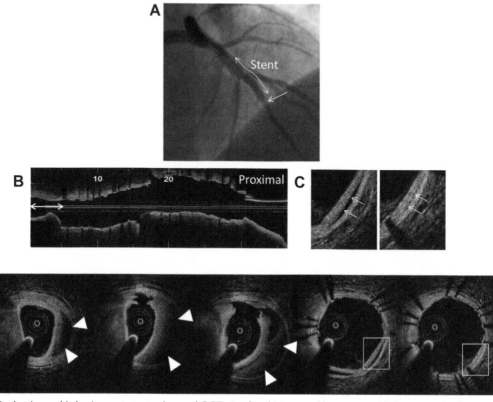

Fig. 8. Angiographic haziness at stent edge and OCT-visualized intramural hematoma. (A) Poststent, haziness can be observed at the distal stent edge on angiography (arrow). (B) Longitudinal image of the stent and distal reference segments with luminal narrowing in the distal reference (double-headed arrow). (C) Magnification of D, delineating that the dissection plane is located within the media (arrows). (D) Consecutive cross-sectional images with the corresponding distal stent edge (double-headed arrow in B) and an intramural hematoma (triangles).

site, and contains a hematoma. To evaluate the severity of a dissection, one should analyze (1) dissection depth (intimal or medial), (2) angle of the dissection flap, (3) residual effective lumen area inside of the dissection flap, and (4) the longitudinal length of the dissection flap (**Fig. 7**). **Fig. 8** shows an example of angiographic haziness at the stent edge in which OCT imaging identified an intramural hematoma.

Chamié and colleagues[18] evaluated 249 post-stent lesions by OCT, and stent edge dissections were found in 37.8% of lesions, most of which (84%) were not visible on angiography. The dissections identified by OCT and angiography were longer, had larger flaps, and had deeper vessel injury than dissections seen only by OCT. Morphologic predictors of dissection were the presence of atherosclerotic plaque at stent edges, calcification angle, fibrous cap thickness, and vessel overstretching defined by stent area/reference lumen area. In this cohort additional stents were implanted in 22.6% of lesions per operator discretion, and 1-year outcomes were similar in lesions with versus without dissection.

SUMMARY

OCT evaluation poststenting includes stent expansion, stent–vessel wall malapposition, tissue (thrombus or plaque) protrusion through stent struts, and dissection. These are precise and reproducible and, therefore, allow careful comparison with subsequent clinical outcomes.

REFERENCES

1. Doi H, Maehara A, Mintz GS, et al. Impact of post-intervention minimal stent area on 9-month follow-up patency of paclitaxel-eluting stents: an integrated intravascular ultrasound analysis from the TAXUS IV, V, and VI and TAXUS ATLAS Workhorse, Long Lesion, and Direct Stent Trials. JACC Cardiovasc Interv 2009;2:1269–75.
2. Cheneau E, Leborgne L, Mintz GS, et al. Predictors of subacute stent thrombosis: results of a systematic intravascular ultrasound study. Circulation 2003;108:43–7.
3. Fujii K, Carlier SG, Mintz GS, et al. Stent underexpansion and residual reference segment stenosis are related to stent thrombosis after sirolimus-eluting stent implantation: an intravascular ultrasound study. J Am Coll Cardiol 2005;45:995–8.
4. Choi SY, Witzenbichler B, Maehara A, et al. Intravascular ultrasound findings of early stent thrombosis after primary percutaneous intervention in acute myocardial infarction: a Harmonizing Outcomes with Revascularization and Stents in Acute Myocardial Infarction (HORIZONS-AMI) substudy. Circ Cardiovasc Interv 2011;4:239–47.
5. Zhang Y, Farooq V, Garcia-Garcia HM, et al. Comparison of intravascular ultrasound versus angiography-guided drug-eluting stent implantation: a meta-analysis of one randomised trial and ten observational studies involving 19,619 patients. EuroIntervention 2012;8:855–65.
6. Klersy C, Ferlini M, Raisaro A, et al. Use of IVUS guided coronary stenting with drug eluting stent: a systematic review and meta-analysis of randomized controlled clinical trials and high quality observational studies. Int J Cardiol 2013;170:54–63.
7. Jang JS, Song YJ, Kang W, et al. Intravascular ultrasound-guided implantation of drug-eluting stents to improve outcome: a meta-analysis. JACC Cardiovasc Interv 2014;7:233–43.
8. Ahn JM, Kang SJ, Yoon SH, et al. Meta-analysis of outcomes after intravascular ultrasound-guided versus angiography-guided drug-eluting stent implantation in 26,503 patients enrolled in three randomized trials and 14 observational studies. Am J Cardiol 2014;113:1338–47.
9. Di Vito L, Yoon JH, Kato K, et al. Comprehensive overview of definitions for optical coherence tomography-based plaque and stent analyses. Coron Artery Dis 2014;25:172–85.
10. Tearney GJ, Regar E, Akasaka T, et al. Consensus standards for acquisition, measurement, and reporting of intravascular optical coherence tomography studies: a report from the international working group for intravascular optical coherence tomography standardization and validation. J Am Coll Cardiol 2012;59:1058–72.
11. Prati F, Guagliumi G, Mintz GS, et al. Expert review document on methodology, terminology, and clinical applications of optical coherence tomography: physical principles, methodology of image acquisition, and clinical application for assessment of coronary arteries and atherosclerosis. Eur Heart J 2010;31:401–15.
12. Tahara S, Bezerra HG, Baibars M, et al. In vitro validation of new Fourier-domain optical coherence tomography. EuroIntervention 2011;6:875–82.
13. Okamura T, Onuma Y, Garcia-Garcia HM, et al. First-in-man evaluation of intravascular optical frequency domain imaging (OFDI) of Terumo: a comparison with intravascular ultrasound and quantitative coronary angiography. EuroIntervention 2011;6:1037–45.
14. Jamil Z, Tearney G, Bruining N, et al. Interstudy reproducibility of the second generation, Fourier domain optical coherence tomography in patients with coronary artery disease and comparison with intravascular ultrasound: a study applying automated contour detection. Int J Cardiovasc Imaging 2013;29:39–51.

15. Bezerra HG, Attizzani GF, Sirbu V, et al. Optical coherence tomography versus intravascular ultrasound to evaluate coronary artery disease and percutaneous coronary intervention. JACC Cardiovasc Interv 2013;6:228–36.

16. Kubo T, Akasaka T, Shite J, et al. Optical coherence tomography compared to intravascular ultrasound in coronary lesion assessment study: OPUS-CLASS study. JACC Cardiovasc Imaging 2013;6: 1095–104.

17. Gonzalo N, Serruys PW, Okamura T, et al. Optical coherence tomography assessment of the acute effects of stent implantation on the vessel wall: a systematic quantitative approach. Heart 2009;95: 1913–9.

18. Chamié D, Bezerra HG, Attizzani GF, et al. Incidence, predictors, morphological characteristics, and clinical outcomes of stent edge dissections detected by optical coherence tomography. JACC Cardiovasc Interv 2013;6:800–13.

19. Im E, Kim BK, Ko YG, et al. Incidences, predictors, and clinical outcomes of acute and late stent malapposition detected by optical coherence tomography after drug-eluting stent implantation. Circ Cardiovasc Interv 2014;7:88–96.

20. Kawamori H, Shite J, Shinke T, et al. Natural consequence of post-intervention stent malapposition, thrombus, tissue prolapse, and dissection assessed by optical coherence tomography at mid-term follow-up. Eur Heart J Cardiovasc Imaging 2013; 14:865–75.

21. Shimamura K, Kubo T, Akasaka T, et al. Outcomes of everolimus-eluting stent incomplete stent apposition: a serial optical coherence tomography analysis. Eur Heart J Cardiovasc Imaging 2015;16: 23–8.

22. Fedele S, Biondi-Zoccai G, Kwiatkowski P, et al. Reproducibility of coronary optical coherence tomography for lumen and length measurements in humans (The CLI-VAR [Centro per la Lotta contro l'Infarto-VARiability] study). Am J Cardiol 2012; 15(110):1106–12.

23. Liu Y, Shimamura K, Kubo T, et al. Comparison of longitudinal geometric measurement in human coronary arteries between frequency-domain optical coherence tomography and intravascular ultrasound. Int J Cardiovasc Imaging 2014;30:271–7.

24. McPherson JA, Maehara A, Weisz G, et al. Residual plaque burden in patients with acute coronary syndromes after successful percutaneous coronary intervention. JACC Cardiovasc Imaging 2012;5: S76–85.

25. Sawada T, Shite J, Negi N, et al. Factors that influence measurements and accurate evaluation of stent apposition by optical coherence tomography. Assessment using a phantom model. Circ J 2009; 73:1841–7.

26. Prati F, Di Vito L, Biondi-Zoccai G, et al. Angiography alone versus angiography plus optical coherence tomography to guide decision-making during percutaneous coronary intervention: the Centro per la Lotta contro l'Infarto-Optimisation of Percutaneous Coronary Intervention (CLI-OPCI) study. EuroIntervention 2012;8:823–9.

27. Habara M, Nasu K, Terashima M, et al. Impact of frequency-domain optical coherence tomography guidance for optimal coronary stent implantation in comparison with intravascular ultrasound guidance. Circ Cardiovasc Interv 2012;5:193–201.

28. Kubo T, Yamano T, Liu Y, et al. Feasibility of optical coronary tomography in quantitative measurement of coronary arteries with lipid-rich plaque. Circ J 2015;79:600–6.

29. Guo N, Maehara A, Mintz GS, et al. Incidence, mechanisms, predictors, and clinical impact of acute and late stent malapposition after primary intervention in patients with acute myocardial infarction: an intravascular ultrasound substudy of the Harmonizing Outcomes with Revascularization and Stents in Acute Myocardial Infarction (HORIZONS-AMI) trial. Circulation 2010;122:1077–84.

30. Steinberg DH, Mintz GS, Mandinov L, et al. Long-term impact of routinely detected early and late incomplete stent apposition: an integrated intravascular ultrasound analysis of the TAXUS IV, V, and VI and TAXUS ATLAS Workhorse, long lesion, and direct stent studies. JACC Cardiovasc Interv 2010;3:486–94.

31. Maehara A, Mintz GS, Lansky AJ, et al. Volumetric intravascular ultrasound analysis of paclitaxel-eluting and bare metal stents in acute myocardial infarction: the harmonizing outcomes with revascularization and stents in acute myocardial infarction intravascular ultrasound substudy. Circulation 2009;120:1875–82.

32. Sugiyama T, Kimura S, Akiyama D, et al. Quantitative assessment of tissue prolapse on optical coherence tomography and its relation to underlying plaque morphologies and clinical outcome in patients with elective stent implantation. Int J Cardiol 2014;176:182–90.

33. Onuma Y, Thuesen L, van Geuns RJ, et al. Randomized study to assess the effect of thrombus aspiration on flow area in patients with ST-elevation myocardial infarction: an optical frequency domain imaging study—TROFI trial. Eur Heart J 2013;34:1050–60.

34. Prati F, Capodanno D, Pawlowski T, et al. Local delivery versus intracoronary infusion of abciximab in patients with acute coronary syndromes. JACC Cardiovasc Interv 2010;3:928–34.

35. Parodi G, Valenti R, Migliorini A, et al. Comparison of manual thrombus aspiration with rheolytic thrombectomy in acute myocardial infarction. Circ Cardiovasc Interv 2013;6:224–30.

Diagnosis and Evaluation of Stent Thrombosis with Optical Coherence Tomography

Alessio Mattesini, MD, Benedetta Bellandi, MD,
Serafina Valente, MD, Guido Parodi, MD, PhD, FESC*

KEYWORDS

- Stent thrombosis • OCT • Intravascular imaging • PCI

KEY POINTS

- Malapposition and stent underexpansion have been identified as predictors of stent thrombosis (ST) that can be evaluated by optical coherence tomography (OCT) at the time of stent implantation to reduce the risk of subsequent ST.
- During follow-up, OCT may identify high-risk intrastent morphology such as neoatherosclerosis.
- OCT-guided management seems to be a feasible, safe, and appropriate approach to assess the efficacy of coronary thrombus removal and to detect the prevalent stent-related factor that caused the ST.
- Owing to the multifactorial nature of ST and the heavy contribution of platelets to the acute event, intracoronary imaging and platelet reactivity evaluation may help to fully understand the cause of ST.

INTRODUCTION

Percutaneous coronary intervention (PCI) with stent implantation is an effective invasive strategy for the treatment of coronary artery disease. The most feared complication related to coronary stent placement is stent thrombosis (ST). This complication is relatively rare, particularly with second-generation drug-eluting stents (DES), occurring in 0.5% to 1% of patients within 1 year after then procedure. When it does occur, ST is associated with substantial morbidity and mortality. It most commonly presents as acute myocardial infarction (MI)[1] requiring emergent repeat PCI with optimal reperfusion occurring only in two-thirds of patients.[2] As a result, ST has been associated with high 30-day mortality rates (range, 25%–30%) as well as with high rates of recurrent ST. In fact, about 20% of patients with a first episode of ST experience a recurrence within 2 years. The mechanisms underlying ST are multifactorial, including patient, procedural and postprocedural treatment characteristics. By virtue of its high resolution and the characteristics of imaging with light, optical coherence tomography (OCT) represents a unique tool for ST diagnosis. Moreover, it can be used to improve the understanding of the particular mechanism of ST in a particular patient, and may thereby guide the most appropriate intervention. Moreover, when used as guidance for complex PCI procedures, OCT may play a role in minimizing the risk of ST. In this review, we provide an update on ST with a particular focus on OCT for its diagnosis and prevention.

DEFINITION AND CLASSIFICATION OF STENT THROMBOSIS

The lack of consensus on the definition of ST among clinical trials has led to disparities in

The authors have no disclosure to declare related to this article.
Department of Cardiology, Careggi Hospital, Largo Brambilla n 3, Florence 50100, Italy
* Corresponding author. Department of Cardiology, Careggi Hospital, Viale Pieraccini 17, Florence I-50134, Italy.
E-mail address: parodiguido@gmail.com

reports of ST and, in particular, has prevented comparison of the rates of ST between studies. To address this issue, the Academic Research Consortium definition of ST has been established.[3] In this definition, ST is categorized currently according to the timing after initial PCI and the objective evidence of ST.

Timing of Stent Thrombosis

ST is considered to be acute when occurring between 0 and 24 hours after stent implantation; subacute between 24 hours and 30 days; late between 30 days and 1 year; and very late after 1 year. The term 'early' ST can also be used to refer to acute and subacute ST.

Definite Stent Thrombosis

Definite ST requires the presence of an angiographic confirmation of ST (the presence of a thrombus that originates in the stent or in the segment 5 mm proximal or distal to the stent) and must be associated with at least 1 of the following criteria within a 48-hour window: acute onset of ischemic symptoms at rest, new ischemic electrocardiographic changes that suggest acute ischemia or typical increase and decrease in cardiac biomarkers, or the presence of a pathologic confirmation of ST (evidence of recent thrombus within the stent determined at autopsy or via examination of tissue retrieved after thrombectomy). The incidental angiographic documentation of stent occlusion in the absence of clinical signs or symptoms is not considered a confirmed ST (silent occlusion).

Probable Stent Thrombosis

Probable ST is defined as the presence of any unexplained death within the first 30 days after stent implantation, or in the presence of any MI related to documented acute ischemia in the territory of the implanted stent without angiographic confirmation of ST and in the absence of any other obvious cause, irrespective of the time after the index procedure.

Possible Stent Thrombosis

Possible ST is defined as any unexplained death from 30 days after stenting until the end of follow-up.

PATHOPHYSIOLOGY OF STENT THROMBOSIS

The pathophysiology of ST is complex and involves several different factors. Platelet function and platelet reactivity on antiplatelet therapy, coagulation factors, and inflammation play a pivotal role in the mechanism of ST. In addition to these elements, ST can be triggered by patient clinical characteristics and risk factors such as the following:

- Chronic renal failure;
- Diabetes;
- Left ventricular dysfunction or type of stent implanted (bare metal stent, first- or second-generation DES, biovascular scaffold);
- Treated lesion characteristics (long, complex lesion, bifurcation, chronic total occlusion);
- Acuity of the index clinical syndrome preceding stenting (stable angina, unstable angina, non-ST elevation MI or ST-elevation MI);
- Procedure-related factors; and
- Other unknown factors (Box 1).[1,4,5]

Different temporal pathophysiologic mechanisms are involved in each category of ST (acute, subacute, late, and very late). Procedure- and mechanical-related factors seem to play a major role in acute/subacute ST, whereas impaired reendothelization, stent malapposition or fracture, hypersensitivity reaction to the polymer used in DES, inflammation, or de novo plaque rupture have important roles in late and very late ST (Box 2).[6,7] It is currently unknown what extent of lack of stent coverage can be considered unsafe. Effective dual antiplatelet therapy is able to mitigate the early risk related to uncovered stent struts. Early discontinuation of dual antiplatelet therapy, as described in the Mechanism Of Stent Thrombosis (MOST) study, or ineffective platelet inhibition owing to poor responsiveness to therapy[8,9] allows the uncovered metallic stent strut to trigger the thrombotic event.[10] The number of uncovered stent struts is a chronic trigger factor, requiring activated platelets to develop thrombosis. Taking into consideration the small amount of available data, it seems that, in the case of a slight lack of stent strut coverage, the occurrence of ST can be provoked by concomitant high on-treatment platelet reactivity, especially when associated with nonresponsiveness to aspirin therapy.[11] Tailored antiplatelet therapy based on platelet function test results was investigated in the Assessment by Double Randomization of a Conventional Antiplatelet Strategy versus a Monitoring-guided Strategy for Drug-Eluting Stent Implantation and of Treatment Interruption versus Continuation One Year after Stenting (ARTIC) and Gauging Responsiveness with A VerifyNow Assay - Impact on Thrombosis And Safety (GRAVITAS) trials showed

Box 1
Patient, lesion, and pharmacologic predictors of stent thrombosis

Patient-related factors
- Diabetes mellitus
- Chronic kidney disease
- Impaired left systolic ventricular function
- Percutaneous coronary intervention for acute coronary syndrome
- Malignancies
- Saphenous venous graft disease

Lesion-related factors
- Diffuse coronary disease with long stent segments
- Small vessel disease
- Bifurcation disease
- Chronic total occlusion disease
- Thrombus containing lesion (stent deployment in necrotic core)

Procedural/stent-related factors
- Stent type (bare metal stent, drug-eluting stents, first- and second-generation drug-eluting stents, bioresorbable vascular scaffold)
- Adjunctive therapeutic agents (paclitaxel, sirolimus, everolimus, zotarolimus)
- Stent polymer (biocompatibility/thrombogenicity)
- Stent design/struts thickness
- Stent length, number
- Covered stent
- Inadequate stent expansion
- Stent undersizing
- Stent malapposition (acute and late)
- Significant inflow or outflow lesions of the stented segments
- Edge dissection limiting inflow or outflow
- Delayed or incomplete endothelization of stent struts
- Hypersensitivity/inflammatory and/or thrombotic reactions to drug-eluting stent polymer
- Strut fractures
- Plaque protrusion
- Development of neoatherosclerosis within stent with new plaque rupture

Pharmacologic factors
- Type and duration of antiplatelet therapy
- Patient-specific response to therapy
- Compliance with antiplatelet therapy

no differences in clinical outcomes, suggesting that the presence of on-treatment reactivity on clopidogrel treatment is only a partially modifiable risk factor,[12–14] although limitations of trial design may have also contributed to these findings.[15] Prasugrel and ticagrelor, which are more powerful $P2Y_{12}$ platelet receptor inhibitors that have a faster onset of action than clopidogrel, significantly reduce ST rates in patients compared with clopidogrel in patients with moderate-to-high risk acute coronary syndrome, suggesting that effective and strong platelet inhibition is associated with a lower rate of ST.[16,17]

Acute/subacute stent thrombosis

Procedure-related and mechanical-related
factors

- Residual target lesion thrombus
- Dissection
- Abnormal blood flow in the stented segment
- Stent underexpansion
- Incomplete stent strut coverage in association
  with high on treatment platelet reactivity
- Combination of the above factors

Late/very late stent thrombosis

- Impaired reendothelization
- Incomplete and or abnormal healing
- Inadequate neointimal stent strut coverage
  stent malapposition or fracture
- Hypersensitivity reaction to the polymer used
  in drug-eluting stent
- Inflammation
- Neoatherosclerosis   development   and
  complications

PROGNOSIS OF STENT THROMBOSIS

ST, especially occurring late, has been a major concern with first-generation DES. Several studies and metaanalyses demonstrated an increased risk of late ST and MI in patients treated with first-generation DES after discontinuation of dual antiplatelet therapy[18] and a steady accrual of ST at a rate of 0.6% to 1% per year, with no evidence of plateau after 4-year follow-up.[19,20] In view of the rare incidence of ST with bare metal stents (BMS), several analyses were performed to address the safety of first-generation DES.[21–24] These studies consistently established that there was not a significant difference of MI and death between first-generation DES and BMS, despite a higher incidence of ST with DES over time. Therefore, the US Food and Drug Administration finally concluded with an advisory suggesting that DES were associated with an higher late incidence of ST compared with BMS, but they were recognized as safe and effective when used for on-label indications.[25]

Second-generation DES, with advanced stent design features such as thinner struts and more compatible biopolymer or bioabsorbable polymers, have been effective at reducing the incidence of ST. Second-generation DES, especially cobalt–chromium alloy everolimus eluting stents have undergone extensive investigation in clinical randomized trials and real-world registries.[26,27] Direct comparison between the different types of second-generation DES, first-generation DES, and BMS is challenging, especially considering the wide range of indications for stent implantation (from stable coronary disease to acute coronary syndromes). Indirect comparisons, through large network metaanalyses, seem to show a significant reduction in ST with second-generation DES compared with either first-generation DES or BMS.[28–30] The reduction of ST rate may carry an important impact on prognosis especially among high-risk patients such as ST-segment elevation MI (STEMI) patients. In this subgroup, cobalt–chromium alloy everolimus eluting stents were associated with significantly lower rates of 1-year cardiac death/MI, MI, definite ST, and definite/probable ST than BMS, whereas DES were associated with significantly lower rates of cardiac death/MI than BMS.[28] The interpretation of these network metaanalyses must incorporate the methodologic limitations of the indirect comparisons.

Even with newer generation DES, ST remains an uncommon but still potentially life-threatening complication after PCI with 10% to 20% mortality at 1 year.[31–33] In a recent study by Armstrong and colleagues, ST-related mortality was significantly higher (9.5%) in early ST compared with late (3.8%) and very late ST (3.6%; *P*<.001). This lower mortality for late and very late ST persisted after multivariable adjustment (odds ratio, 0.53 [95% CI, 0.36–0.79] and 0.58 [95% CI, 0.43–0.79], respectively).

ST remains an issue with the new everolimus-eluting bioresorbable vascular scaffold (ABSORB BVS, Abbott, Santa Clara, CA). In the large GHOST (Gauging coronary Healing with biO-resorbable Scaffolding plaTforms in Europe) retrospective, multicenter European registry, the cumulative incidence of definite/probable scaffold thrombosis was 1.5% at 30 days and 2.1% at 6 months, with 16 of 23 cases occurring within the first 30 days after BVS implantation. A large proportion of STs occurred despite ongoing dual antiplatelet therapy. ST resulted in cardiac death in 3 of 23 patients (13%) and nonfatal reinfarction in 15 of 23 cases (65%). ST occurred acutely (within 24 hours) in 5 of 23 (22%) patients, subacutely (after 24 hours but within 1 month after implantation) in 11 of 23 patients (48%), and late (after 30 days) in 7 of

23 patients (30%). The median time to occurrence of early (acute or subacute) ST was 5 days (interquartile range, 0–9).[34]

TREATMENT OF STENT THROMBOSIS

The clinical presentation of a coronary ST is very often an ST-elevation MI. According to the current guidelines, the preferred treatment option should be primary PCI, as in the case of de novo STEMI owing to occlusive thrombus complicating an atherosclerotic plaque. Primary PCI has been shown to be effective in the recanalization of the infarct-related artery of patients with STEMI owing to ST. An optimal result was obtained in 96% of cases, without difference compared with patients with de novo STEMI.[10] Because primary PCI for treatment of ST seems to mirror the results of primary PCI in the setting of a primary coronary event, it should be considered the therapy of choice in this subgroup of patients with STEMI. Poor results after balloon angioplasty alone or intracoronary fibrinolysis are described in literature. The use of glyocoprotein IIb/IIIa inhibitors during primary PCI for ST, in particular intracoronary abciximab, is described in small studies that suggest a clinical benefit.[35–37] The choice between rheolytic thrombectomy or manual thrombus aspiration may be performed in relation to thrombotic burden, availability, and operator experience. Additional stenting technique may be considered in the presence of significant residual thrombosis, dissection, neointimal hyperplasia, plaque prolapse, or edge progression, as well as with stent fracture. In some cases, wire crossing of the thrombotic occlusion was able to dissolve the majority of the fresh thrombotic burden and the intervention was concluded with balloon dilation of the previously implanted stent. As documented by the long procedural and fluoroscopic times and by the relevant contrast medium amount used, primary PCI for ST is generally a complex procedure. In patients with ST, the contrast media amount may lead to an increased risk of contrast-induced nephropathy, as suggested by the higher creatinine value after PCI compared with patients with de novo STEMI. Poor outcome of patients with ST was attributed mainly to the suboptimal PCI result (TIMI [final coronary Thrombolysis In Myocardial Infarction] grade 3 flow in only 80% of patients). Despite immediate and effective mechanical infarct-related artery recanalization, patients with ST develop a large MI; ST is associated with a poor outcome independent of a patient's risk profile, and recurrence of ST is common.

More aggressive management seems justified in this subgroup of patients with STEMI; therefore, achievement of an optimal primary PCI result in this subset of patients with STEMI is important. In fact, the lack of an optimal PCI result emerged as an independent predictor of adverse events.[38]

Antiplatelet therapy is a cornerstone in acute coronary syndrome, in particular in ST setting. ST has a multifactorial pathophysiology and platelet function plays a pivotal role; therefore, platelet function tests have a rational use in this subset of patients. Platelet function tests should be performed before glycoprotein IIb/IIIa inhibitors (GPI) use and they are useful also to evaluate patient's compliance with antiplatelet therapy. In the case of high on-treatment reactivity on $P2Y_{12}$ inhibitors, treatment optimization is strongly encouraged (see **Fig. 3**).[38–40]

OPTICAL COHERENCE TOMOGRAPHY–GUIDED STENT DEPLOYMENT

In the past 2 decades, intravascular ultrasound (IVUS) has been used to guide stent deployment and to assess the result after stent implantation. IVUS criteria, based on a combination of lumen area, diameter, and comparison of the minimal luminal area within the stent with the reference area proximal and distal, were proposed to guide the optimization of stent deployment.[41,42] With IVUS, the echogenicity of stent struts and difficulty in defining the luminal contours may complicate the assessment of lumen area, especially when the lumen geometry is not fully circular. Specific OCT criteria for optimal stent deployment assessment have not been defined, but OCT is certainly adequate to assess stent deployment based on the lumen criteria. In fact, owing to the low penetration of OCT, quantification of the total vessel diameter from the external elastic lamina is often impractical and may be limited to a minority of distal reference segments with small amount of fibrotic or fibrocalcified plaque. No clinical head-to-head studies have yet compared the feasibility or clinical outcomes of IVUS and OCT. However, the ability of OCT to address luminal areas and identify underexpansion, malapposition, uneven stent strut distribution, or small intrastent thrombotic formations makes the technique an attractive tool for the optimization of stent implantation to prevent mechanical complications that may result in ST. OCT studies based on sequential analysis also showed that incomplete stent apposition after deployment correlate with delayed neointimal coverage.[43] Struts are defined as being malapposed when the distance between the strut and luminal surfaces is greater than the strut's thickness, including the thickness of the polymer for DES.[44] Acute malapposition can contribute to ST by disturbing the normal laminar blood flow along the vessel wall, and promoting the deposition of platelets and fibrin.[45] In the case of the thick-strutted BVS, malapposition of the stent might create a higher grade of flow disturbance and abnormal shear stress compared with that which occurs from malapposition of the thin struts of a second-generation DES.

Optical Coherence Tomography and Bifurcation Lesions

Lesions located at a vessel bifurcation represent a challenging lesion subset, with relatively high rates of acute and late stent failure, even in the DES era.[46] IVUS can be used for optimal sizing of the main and side branch vessels, identification of plaque location and characteristics before stent deployment, and for optimization of procedural results.[47] OCT can assess the same quantitative parameters of bifurcation segments obtained with IVUS[48]; however, its particular usefulness consists in the detection of strut apposition and procedural guidance to optimize it. Tyczynski and colleagues[49] demonstrated that the rate of malapposed struts was significantly higher at the side branch ostium than in the vessel side opposite to the ostium in both simple (1 stent) or complex strategies for bifurcation stenting. In a larger series of bifurcation lesions, Viceconte and colleagues[50] observed a persistent malapposition rates as high as 43% despite consistent use of proximal optimization technique and kissing balloon dilatation.

Bench tests made in coronary phantoms have demonstrated that the position where the guidewire recrosses the stent struts into the side branch is among the most important elements influencing stent cell opening and strut apposition in the side branch after balloon dilatation. Angiography and IVUS are inadequate to detect the site of wire recrossing. The superior resolution of OCT makes this technique ideal for guiding stent recrossing in bifurcations. Alegria-Barrero and colleagues[51] analyzed the feasibility and effectiveness of OCT-guided stent recrossing compared with angiographic guidance in which OCT was used only for documentary purposes. Among a population of 52 patients, the OCT-guided group (12 patients) showed a significantly lower number of malapposed stent struts, especially in the quadrants toward the side branch ostium

(9.5% vs 42.3%; $P<.001$). Although OCT guidance seems to improve mechanical characteristics associated with ST, larger clinical studies are required to assess whether bifurcation optimization under OCT guidance leads to a clinical benefit in terms of the rates of ST and restenosis.[52]

Stent Edges

Landing zone and stent edges are another pivotal point for PCI technical success, because stent edges could be underexpanded and thrombus, plaque shift, or dissections may occur after stent implantation. OCT can display accurately the morphology of the proximal and distal stent edge and any complications. OCT has a higher sensitivity compared with angiography for the detection of edge dissections.[53] It is important, however, not to overreact to small thin mobile dissections (better called flails), which have a very low likelihood of leading to vessel closure.[53] Furthermore, the composition of the plaque where the stent edge will land should be carefully taken into account, because PCI when a stent edge is implanted within a lipid pool is associated with a significantly higher rate of postprocedural MI.[54]

OPTICAL COHERENCE TOMOGRAPHY AND STENT FOLLOW-UP

OCT has been validated for the evaluation of strut coverage and neointimal response with an accuracy resembling that of histology.[55,56] Delayed healing and poor endothelialization are common findings in pathologic specimens of vessels treated with DES[57,58] and recent pathologic studies demonstrated that the best predictor of late ST is the ratio of uncovered/total stent struts.[59,60] BMS develop circumferential coverage with an average thickness of 500 μm or more, which are well-visualized with IVUS and angiography. DES delay and prevent the neointimal response so that the average late lumen loss can be less than 100 μm. This amount of intimal thickening is not detectable with IVUS because of its limited axial resolution and the presence of artifacts around stent struts,[61] but can be detected by OCT, which provides 10 to 30 times higher resolution. Several experimental and clinical studies have demonstrated a high correlation between OCT and histologic measurements of neointimal coverage of stent struts.[55,62] OCT analysis of strut coverage has improved the understanding of the vascular healing process in different vessel anatomies. Impaired neointimal coverage is associated more frequently with nonapposed side branch struts and incomplete stent apposition compared with well-apposed struts. A greater distance of the strut surface from the vessel wall (ie, more severe malapposition), is associated more frequently with uncovered struts.[63,64]

Several studies suggest a close relation between OCT patterns of in-stent restenosis and histology.[65] Different light attenuation and backscattering intensity may reveal the presence of heterogeneous components in the neointimal tissue.[65–67] Homogeneous signals are associated with fibrotic tissue, as found in early BMS restenotic hyperplasia. Heterogeneous patterns can be caused by immature, early intimal changes (eg, proteoglycans and fibrin accumulation) or by neoatherosclerosis. Although the most frequent clinical presentation of neointimal hyperplasia is stable angina, in-stent neoatherosclerosis seems to be associated with acute coronary syndromes.[68] Therefore, OCT might play a pivotal role in the guidance of treatment of in-stent restenosis.

DIAGNOSIS OF STENT THROMBOSIS BY OPTICAL COHERENCE TOMOGRAPHY

Coronary angiography is accepted as the gold standard imaging technique for coronary intervention. The identification of ST at angiogram is required for the Academic Research Consortium definition of definite ST. However, angiography may easily miss small or moderate-sized thrombi. OCT is ideally suited for the evaluation of ST, given its high resolution, excellent contrast between the vessel lumen and other intravascular structures, and the typical appearance seen with thrombi. At OCT analysis, red blood cell–rich "red" thrombus can be identified by high backscattering and signal-free shadowing protrusion, whereas platelet-rich "white" thrombus is depicted as signal-rich, low backscattering mass projecting into the lumen (Figs. 1 and 2). However, a mixed thrombus with intermediate features is often observed. In a study by Kume and colleagues,[69] OCT was able to differentiate between "red" and "white" thrombi with high sensitivity (90%) and specificity (88%) The main limit of OCT is to distinguish between in-stent plaque prolapse, thrombus protrusion, and acute ST. However, this issue is mainly limited to OCT performed immediately after deployment of a stent in soft lesions with a large thrombus burden. At long term follow-up, OCT can discern between in-stent restenosis owing to neointimal hyperplasia and neoatherosclerotic with or without superimposed thrombus.

MANAGEMENT OF STENT THROMBOSIS USING OPTICAL COHERENCE TOMOGRAPHY

PCI for ST is often a challenging and technically demanding procedure. There are 2 key points for procedural success: first, the identification

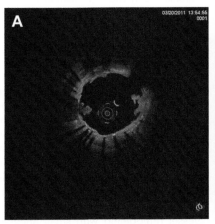 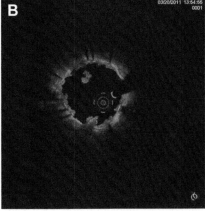

Fig. 1. Subacute stent thrombosis in a patient with anterior acute myocardial infarction (ST-segment elevation myocardial infarction) treated 4 days before with everolimus drug-eluting stent implantation and receiving clopidogrel maintenance therapy. The patient displayed high on-treatment reactivity at the time of stent thrombosis. Images show the presence of fresh thrombus, characterized by homogeneous signal-rich structure without backscattering. After manual thrombus aspiration residual thrombus burden was limited within the stent by optical coherence tomography (OCT). (A, B) Adequate stent apposition and initial strut coverage were evident, suggesting no need for repeated thrombectomy, stent overexpansion, or additional stenting. The patient was treated with intracoronary abciximab and switched from clopidogrel to prasugrel.

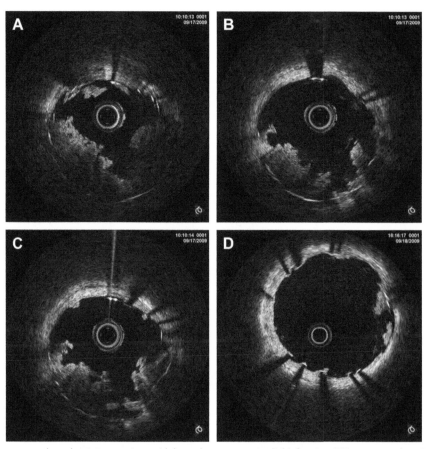

Fig. 2. Acute stent thrombosis in a patient with lateral acute myocardial infarction (ST-segment elevation myocardial infarction [STEMI]) treated during primary drug-eluting stent implantation with bivalirudin and a 600-mg clopidogrel loading dose 22 hours before stent thrombosis. The young woman was a carrier of the CYP2C19*2 polymorphism. (A–D) After manual thrombus aspiration, residual thrombosis was evident within the stent by optical coherence tomography, suggesting the need for repeated thrombectomy and implementation of antithrombotic therapy.

or exclusion of a procedurally related mechanism potentially involved in stent failure, and second the optimization of antiplatelet treatment on the basis of platelet reactivity. The 2 management processes should run parallel once the angiographic diagnosis of definite ST has been made (Fig. 3).

Although there are few data available regarding the optimal interventional strategy for ST, in our daily clinical practice, manual thrombus aspiration is the first step when facing a totally occlusive ST.[70] In case of vessel recanalization with sufficient contrast medium runoff, OCT can be performed to assess whether an underlying mechanism of stent failure is detectable. Stent underexpansion and severe strut malapposition are probably the most frequent procedural mechanism leading to ST. Prompt identification and correction of these conditions are mandatory to prevent ST recurrence. The clinical impact of

limited edge dissections visualized with OCT after stent deployment is unknown. However, the identification of significant edge dissection underlying ST is pivotal to guide the procedure because the deployment of an additional stent is generally required. OCT also enables the assessment of residual thrombus burden after thrombus aspiration. When a large amount of material is still present, further thrombectomy attempts would seem to be reasonable.

OCT is also able to demonstrate the pathologic healing process related to ST.[71] Positive vessel remodeling with small aneurysm formation is known to be associated with first generation DES. OCT, by highlighting this condition, may play a role in procedural decision making (ie, in-stent deployment of a second-generation DES or covered stent, antiplatelet treatment optimization). In-stent neoatherosclerosis has been also described with OCT as a possible

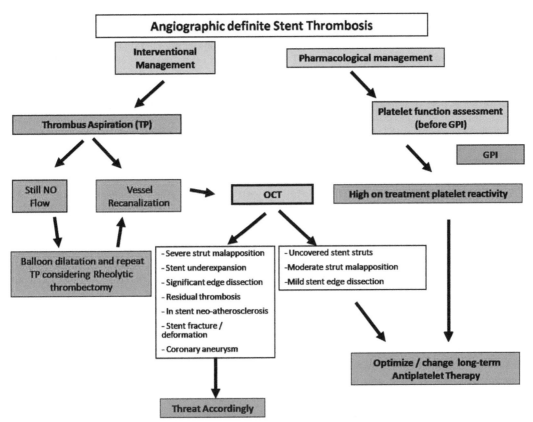

Fig. 3. Proposed diagnostic–therapeutic flowchart for the management of definite stent thrombosis using optical coherence tomography (OCT). GPI, glycoprotein IIb/IIIa inhibitors.

stent restenosis pattern.[72,73] Indeed, this pathologic healing pattern, which is frequently characterized by the presence of multiple thin cap fibroatheroma, is related to a high risk of ST. Even if there are not specific recommendations for the treatment of ST in this specific circumstance, its identification is pivotal to shed light on the mechanism of stent failure.

ST may also be related to ineffective antiplatelet therapy. Along with interventional management, platelet reactivity should be assessed in the catheterization laboratory before the possible administration of glycoprotein IIb/IIIa inhibitors to identify this risk factor, because high on-treatment reactivity on clopidogrel therapy has been associated with ST. Identification of noncompliance or high on-treatment reactivity may inform the selection of more potent P2Y$_{12}$ inhibitors, particularly whether a mechanical condition possibly explaining ST is not identified by OCT.

PREVENTION OF STENT THROMBOSIS

Understanding the pathophysiology and the factors triggering ST is the cornerstone to prevent it. Patient selection is the first step for preventing ST which is known to occur more frequently in complex patients and lesions, particularly in those with acute coronary syndromes, chronic kidney disease, diabetes mellitus and diffuse disease, small vessels, and bifurcation lesions requiring multiple stents.[1,2] Moreover, poor response to clopidogrel is associated with ST and cardiac mortality, and new platelet P2Y$_{12}$ receptor inhibitors should be considered after PCI in acute coronary syndrome patients.[12] Additionally, premature discontinuation of dual antiplatelet therapy within 6 months of the intervention has been associated with a higher incidence of ST especially when the reason for discontinuation is owing to a trauma or the need for operative procedures.[74] Understanding the risk of ST based on these patient-related factors facilitates the use of both procedural and therapeutic strategies aimed to minimize the risk of ST.

Procedural factors associated with ST include the stent-type selected (i.e. BMS or DES, different type of DES, BVS) as well as whether the stent has been optimally deployed. Nakamura and colleagues[75] demonstrated with IVUS that stent underexpansion occurs not infrequently after stent deployment and was associated with ST. These results have been confirmed with OCT in the MOST study.[10] In this study, a smaller minimal in-stent area was associated with an higher incidence of subacute ST (minimal in-stent, 2.1 vs 2.9 mm^2 in ST patients and controls, respectively; $P = .05$). Late and very late ST was associated with a greater distance of malapposition distance at the thrombus site compared with matched controls (0.45 vs 0.12 mm; $P = .019$). Late and very late ST also had a greater percentage of malapposed and uncovered struts compared with matched controls. On the basis of these observations, adequate stent sizing and deployment with prolonged (>10 s) inflation at high pressure (>14 atm) and after dilatation with noncompliant balloons are considered essential to minimize ST, especially in complex and calcific lesions, when stent underexpansion and malapposition may occur more frequently.

Although there are no definitive data, a recent metaanalysis that included a randomized trials and 10 observational studies reported a lower incidence of ST when PCI was performed under IVUS guidance compared with angiography alone.[76] Similarly, in a study using propensity score–matched analysis, patients undergoing IVUS-guided DES implantation had lower definite ST at 30 days and 12 months compared with those who had not received IVUS guidance.[25] Especially in complex lesions, intravascular imaging used for PCI guidance through the different procedural steps (ie, before the intervention, before stenting, and after stent deployment) might be effective to minimize ST.

Currently, there are concerns with regard to the rates of ST with BVS.[34] In our experience, OCT is a cornerstone for guidance of PCI with BVS because it allows for specific lesion preparation, correct vessel sizing and scaffold selection, and meticulous deployment optimization.[77] In a complex series of BVS-treated lesions, use of OCT for optimization enable the achievement postprocedural area stenosis, minimal lumen area, and an eccentricity index similar to that of second-generation DES platforms.[78]

SUMMARY

ST is a complex process with multifactorial causes encompassing stent-specific, procedural, and patient-specific characteristics. Several mechanical factors, such as malapposition and stent underexpansion, have been identified as predictors of ST. These factors can be evaluated comprehensively and accurately by OCT at the time of initial stent implantation in the hope of reducing the risk of subsequent ST. Over follow-up, OCT may identify high-risk intrastent morphology such as neoatherosclerosis. When ST does occur, OCT-guided examination seems to be a feasible, safe, and appropriate approach to assess the efficacy of coronary thrombus removal and to detect the prevalent stent-related factor that caused the ST, thereby informing the optimal interventional approach. Owing to the multifactorial nature of ST and the heavy contribution of platelets to the acute event, intracoronary imaging may be combined with the evaluation of platelet reactivity by platelet function tests to understand fully the cause of ST on a patient-by-patient basis, and thereby establish a tailored interventional and pharmacologic approach.

REFERENCES

1. Holmes DR Jr, Kereiakes DJ, Garg S, et al. Stent thrombosis. J Am Coll Cardiol 2010;56(17):1357–65.
2. Burzotta F, Parma A, Pristipino C, et al. Angiographic and clinical outcome of invasively managed patients with thrombosed coronary bare metal or drug-eluting stents: the OPTIMIST study. Eur Heart J 2008;29(24):3011–21.
3. Cutlip DE, Windecker S, Mehran R, et al. Clinical end points in coronary stent trials: a case for standardized definitions. Circulation 2007;115(17):2344–51.
4. Nakazawa G. Stent thrombosis of drug eluting stent: pathological perspective. J Cardiol 2011;58(2):84–91.
5. Armstrong EJ, Feldman DN, Wang TY, et al. Clinical presentation, management, and outcomes of angiographically documented early, late, and very late stent thrombosis. JACC Cardiovasc Interv 2012;5(2):131–40.
6. Palmerini T, Biondi-Zoccai G, Della Riva D, et al. Stent thrombosis with drug-eluting stents: is the paradigm shifting? J Am Coll Cardiol 2013;62(21):1915–21.
7. Luscher TF, Steffel J, Eberli FR, et al. Drug-eluting stent and coronary thrombosis: biological mechanisms and clinical implications. Circulation 2007;115(8):1051–8.
8. Price MJ, Endemann S, Gollapudi RR, et al. Prognostic significance of post-clopidogrel platelet reactivity assessed by a point-of-care assay on thrombotic events after drug-eluting stent implantation. Eur Heart J 2008;29:992–1000.
9. Stone GW, Witzenbichler B, Weisz G, et al. Platelet reactivity and clinical outcomes after coronary

artery implantation of drug-eluting stents (ADAPT-DES): a prospective multicentre registry study. Lancet 2013;382:614–23.

10. Parodi G, La Manna A, Di Vito L, et al. Stent-related defects in patients presenting with stent thrombosis: differences at optical coherence tomography between subacute and late/very late thrombosis in the Mechanism Of Stent Thrombosis (MOST) study. EuroIntervention 2013;9(8):936–44.

11. Wenaweser P, Hess O. Stent thrombosis is associated with an impaired response to antiplatelet therapy. J Am Coll Cardiol 2005;46(5):CS5–6.

12. Parodi G, Marcucci R, Valenti R, et al. High residual platelet reactivity after clopidogrel loading and long-term cardiovascular events among patients with acute coronary syndromes undergoing PCI. JAMA 2011;306(11):1215–23.

13. Price MJ, Angiolillo DJ, Teirstein PS, et al. Platelet reactivity and cardiovascular outcomes after percutaneous coronary intervention: a time-dependent analysis of the Gauging Responsiveness with a VerifyNow P2Y12 assay: impact on thrombosis and safety (GRAVITAS) trial. Circulation 2011;124(10):1132–7.

14. Collet JP, Cayla G, Cuisset T, et al. Randomized comparison of platelet function monitoring to adjust antiplatelet therapy versus standard of care: rationale and design of the assessment with a double randomization of (1) a fixed dose versus a monitoring-guided dose of aspirin and clopidogrel after DES implantation, and (2) treatment interruption versus continuation, 1 year after stenting (ARCTIC) study. Am Heart J 2011;161(1):5–12.e5.

15. Angiolillo DJ, Ferreiro JL, Price MJ, et al. Platelet function and genetic testing. J Am Coll Cardiol 2013;62:S21–31.

16. Wiviott SD, Trenk D, Frelinger AL, et al. Prasugrel compared with high loading- and maintenance-dose clopidogrel in patients with planned percutaneous coronary intervention: the Prasugrel in comparison to clopidogrel for inhibition of platelet activation and aggregation-thrombolysis in myocardial infarction 44 trial. Circulation 2007;116(25):2923–32.

17. Wallentin L, Becker RC, Budaj A, et al. Ticagrelor versus clopidogrel in patients with acute coronary syndromes. N Engl J Med 2009;361(11):1045–57.

18. Eisenstein EL, Anstrom KJ, Kong DF, et al. Clopidogrel use and long-term clinical outcomes after drug-eluting stent implantation. JAMA 2007;297(2):159–68.

19. Wenaweser P, Daemen J, Zwahlen M, et al. Incidence and correlates of drug-eluting stent thrombosis in routine clinical practice. 4-year results from a large 2-institutional cohort study. J Am Coll Cardiol 2008;52(14):1134–40.

20. Camenzind E, Steg PG, Wijns W. Stent thrombosis late after implantation of first-generation drug-eluting stents: a cause for concern. Circulation 2007;115(11):1440–55 [discussion: 1455].

21. Ellis SG, Colombo A, Grube E, et al. Incidence, timing, and correlates of stent thrombosis with the polymeric paclitaxel drug-eluting stent: a TAXUS II, IV, V, and VI meta-analysis of 3,445 patients followed for up to 3 years. J Am Coll Cardiol 2007;49(10):1043–51.

22. Kastrati A, Mehilli J, Pache J, et al. Analysis of 14 trials comparing sirolimus-eluting stents with bare-metal stents. N Engl J Med 2007;356(10):1030–9.

23. Kolandaivelu K, Swaminathan R, Gibson WJ, et al. Stent thrombogenicity early in high-risk interventional settings is driven by stent design and deployment and protected by polymer-drug coatings. Circulation 2011;123(13):1400–9.

24. Stone GW, Moses JW, Ellis SG, et al. Safety and efficacy of sirolimus- and paclitaxel-eluting coronary stents. N Engl J Med 2007;356(10):998–1008.

25. Popma JJ, Weiner B, Cowley MJ, et al. FDA advisory panel on the safety and efficacy of drug-eluting stents: summary of findings and recommendations. J Interv Cardiol 2007;20(6):425–46.

26. Raber L, Juni P, Nuesch E, et al. Long-term comparison of everolimus-eluting and sirolimus-eluting stents for coronary revascularization. J Am Coll Cardiol 2011;57(21):2143–51.

27. Baber U, Mehran R, Sharma SK, et al. Impact of the everolimus-eluting stent on stent thrombosis: a meta-analysis of 13 randomized trials. J Am Coll Cardiol 2011;58(15):1569–77.

28. Palmerini T, Biondi-Zoccai G, Della Riva D, et al. Clinical outcomes with drug-eluting and bare-metal stents in patients with ST-segment elevation myocardial infarction: evidence from a comprehensive network meta-analysis. J Am Coll Cardiol 2013;62(6):496–504.

29. Palmerini T, Biondi-Zoccai G, Della Riva D, et al. Stent thrombosis with drug-eluting and bare-metal stents: evidence from a comprehensive network meta-analysis. Lancet 2012;379(9824):1393–402.

30. Bangalore S, Toklu B, Amoroso N, et al. Bare metal stents, durable polymer drug eluting stents, and biodegradable polymer drug eluting stents for coronary artery disease: mixed treatment comparison meta-analysis. BMJ 2013;347:f6625.

31. van Werkum JW, Heestermans AA, de Korte FI, et al. Long-term clinical outcome after a first angiographically confirmed coronary stent thrombosis: an analysis of 431 cases. Circulation 2009;119(6):828–34.

32. Kimura T, Morimoto T, Kozuma K, et al. Comparisons of baseline demographics, clinical presentation, and long-term outcome among patients with early, late, and very late stent thrombosis of sirolimus-eluting stents: observations from the

Registry of Stent Thrombosis for Review and Reevaluation (RESTART). Circulation 2010;122(1):52–61.

33. de la Torre Hernandez JM, Alfonso F, Gimeno F, et al. Thrombosis of second-generation drug-eluting stents in real practice results from the multicenter Spanish registry ESTROFA-2 (Estudio Espanol Sobre Trombosis de Stents Farmacoactivos de Segunda Generacion-2). JACC Cardiovasc Interv 2010;3(9):911–9.

34. Capodanno D, Gori T, Nef H, et al. Percutaneous coronary intervention with everolimus-eluting bioresorbable vascular scaffolds in routine clinical practice: early and midterm outcomes from the European multicentre GHOST-EU registry. EuroIntervention 2015;10:1144–53.

35. Hasdai D, Garratt KN, Holmes DR Jr, et al. Coronary angioplasty and intracoronary thrombolysis are of limited efficacy in resolving early intracoronary stent thrombosis. J Am Coll Cardiol 1996;28(2):361–7.

36. Casserly IP, Hasdai D, Berger PB, et al. Usefulness of abciximab for treatment of early coronary artery stent thrombosis. Am J Cardiol 1998;82(8):981–5.

37. Silva JA, White CJ, Ramee SR, et al. Treatment of coronary stent thrombosis with rheolytic thrombectomy: results from a multicenter experience. Catheter Cardiovasc Interv 2003;58(1):11–7.

38. Parodi G, Memisha G, Bellandi B, et al. Effectiveness of primary percutaneous coronary interventions for stent thrombosis. Am J Cardiol 2009;103(7):913–6.

39. Meier P, Zbinden R, Togni M, et al. Coronary collateral function long after drug-eluting stent implantation. J Am Coll Cardiol 2007;49(1):15–20.

40. Rinfret S, Cutlip DE, Katsiyiannis PT, et al. Rheolytic thrombectomy and platelet glycoprotein IIb/IIIa blockade for stent thrombosis. Catheter Cardiovasc Interv 2002;57(1):24–30.

41. de Jaegere P, Mudra H, Figulla H, et al. Intravascular ultrasound-guided optimized stent deployment. Immediate and 6 months clinical and angiographic results from the Multicenter Ultrasound Stenting in Coronaries Study (MUSIC Study). Eur Heart J 1998;19(8):1214–23.

42. Russo RJ, Silva PD, Teirstein PS, et al. A randomized controlled trial of angiography versus intravascular ultrasound-directed bare-metal coronary stent placement (the AVID Trial). Circ Cardiovasc Interv 2009;2(2):113–23.

43. Gutierrez-Chico JL, Wykrzykowska J, Nuesch E, et al. Vascular tissue reaction to acute malapposition in human coronary arteries: sequential assessment with optical coherence tomography. Circ Cardiovasc Interv 2012;5(1):20–9. S1–8.

44. Prati F, Guagliumi G, Mintz GS, et al. Expert review document part 2: methodology, terminology and clinical applications of optical coherence tomography for the assessment of interventional procedures. Eur Heart J 2012;33(20):2513–20.

45. Alfonso F, Suarez A, Perez-Vizcayno MJ, et al. Intravascular ultrasound findings during episodes of drug-eluting stent thrombosis. J Am Coll Cardiol 2007;50(21):2095–7.

46. Foin N, Mattesini A, Ghione M, et al. Tools & techniques clinical: optimising stenting strategy in bifurcation lesions with insights from in vitro bifurcation models. EuroIntervention 2013;9(7):885–7.

47. Suarez de Lezo J, Medina A, Martin P, et al. Predictors of ostial side branch damage during provisional stenting of coronary bifurcation lesions not involving the side branch origin: an ultrasonographic study. EuroIntervention 2012;7(10):1147–54.

48. Di Mario C, Iakovou I, van der Giessen WJ, et al. Optical coherence tomography for guidance in bifurcation lesion treatment. EuroIntervention 2010;6(Suppl J):J99–106.

49. Tyczynski P, Ferrante G, Moreno-Ambroj C, et al. Simple versus complex approaches to treating coronary bifurcation lesions: direct assessment of stent strut apposition by optical coherence tomography. Rev Esp Cardiol 2010;63(8):904–14.

50. Viceconte N, Tyczynski P, Ferrante G, et al. Immediate results of bifurcational stenting assessed with optical coherence tomography. Catheter Cardiovasc Interv 2013;81(3):519–28.

51. Alegria-Barrero E, Foin N, Chan PH, et al. Choosing the right cell: guidance with three-dimensional optical coherence tomography of bifurcational stenting. Eur Heart J Cardiovasc Imaging 2012;13(5):443.

52. Alegria-Barrero E, Foin N, Chan PH, et al. Optical coherence tomography for guidance of distal cell recrossing in bifurcation stenting: choosing the right cell matters. EuroIntervention 2012;8(2):205–13.

53. Gonzalo N, Serruys PW, Okamura T, et al. Relation between plaque type and dissections at the edges after stent implantation: an optical coherence tomography study. Int J Cardiol 2011;150(2):151–5.

54. Imola F, Occhipinti M, Biondi-Zoccai G, et al. Association between proximal stent edge positioning on atherosclerotic plaques containing lipid pools and postprocedural myocardial infarction (from the CLI-POOL Study). Am J Cardiol 2013;111(4):526–31.

55. Prati F, Zimarino M, Stabile E, et al. Does optical coherence tomography identify arterial healing after stenting? An in vivo comparison with histology, in a rabbit carotid model. Heart 2008;94(2):217–21.

56. Murata A, Wallace-Bradley D, Tellez A, et al. Accuracy of optical coherence tomography in the evaluation of neointimal coverage after stent implantation. JACC Cardiovasc Imaging 2010;3(1):76–84.

57. Virmani R, Guagliumi G, Farb A, et al. Localized hypersensitivity and late coronary thrombosis secondary to a sirolimus-eluting stent: should we be cautious? Circulation 2004;109(6):701–5.

58. Joner M, Finn AV, Farb A, et al. Pathology of drug-eluting stents in humans: delayed healing and late thrombotic risk. J Am Coll Cardiol 2006;48(1):193–202.

59. Katoh H, Shite J, Shinke T, et al. Delayed neointimalization on sirolimus-eluting stents: 6-month and 12-month follow up by optical coherence tomography. Circ J 2009;73(6):1033–7.

60. Finn AV, Joner M, Nakazawa G, et al. Pathological correlates of late drug-eluting stent thrombosis: strut coverage as a marker of endothelialization. Circulation 2007;115(18):2435–41.

61. Tanigawa J, Barlis P, Di Mario C. Intravascular optical coherence tomography: optimisation of image acquisition and quantitative assessment of stent strut apposition. EuroIntervention 2007;3(1):128–36.

62. Suzuki Y, Ikeno F, Koizumi T, et al. In vivo comparison between optical coherence tomography and intravascular ultrasound for detecting small degrees of in-stent neointima after stent implantation. JACC Cardiovasc Interv 2008;1(2):168–73.

63. Gutierrez-Chico JL, Regar E, Nuesch E, et al. Delayed coverage in malapposed and side-branch struts with respect to well-apposed struts in drug-eluting stents: in vivo assessment with optical coherence tomography. Circulation 2011;124(5):612–23.

64. Kim BK, Hong MK, Shin DH, et al. Relationship between stent malapposition and incomplete neointimal coverage after drug-eluting stent implantation. J Interv Cardiol 2012;25(3):270–7.

65. Nakano M, Vorpahl M, Otsuka F, et al. Ex vivo assessment of vascular response to coronary stents by optical frequency domain imaging. JACC Cardiovasc Imaging 2012;5(1):71–82.

66. Li QX, Fu QQ, Shi SW, et al. Relationship between plasma inflammatory markers and plaque fibrous cap thickness determined by intravascular optical coherence tomography. Heart 2010;96(3):196–201.

67. Maurovich-Horvat P, Schlett CL, Alkadhi H, et al. Differentiation of early from advanced coronary atherosclerotic lesions: systematic comparison of CT, intravascular US, and optical frequency domain imaging with histopathologic examination in ex vivo human hearts. Radiology 2012;265(2):393–401.

68. Kang SJ, Mintz GS, Akasaka T, et al. Optical coherence tomographic analysis of in-stent neoatherosclerosis after drug-eluting stent implantation. Circulation 2011;123(25):2954–63.

69. Kume T, Okura H, Miyamoto Y, et al. Natural history of stent edge dissection, tissue protrusion and incomplete stent apposition detectable only on optical coherence tomography after stent implantation - preliminary observation. Circ J 2012;76(3):698–703.

70. Migliorini A, Stabile A, Rodriguez AE, et al. Comparison of AngioJet rheolytic thrombectomy before direct infarct artery stenting with direct stenting alone in patients with acute myocardial infarction. The JETSTENT trial. J Am Coll Cardiol 2010;56(16):1298–306.

71. Zivelonghi C, Ghione M, Kilickesmez K, et al. Intracoronary optical coherence tomography: a review of clinical applications. J Cardiovasc Med (Hagerstown) 2014;15(7):543–53.

72. Yang YJ, Kim M, Kim C, et al. Late stent thrombosis after drug-eluting stent implantation: a rare case of accelerated neo-atherosclerosis and early manifestation of neointimal rupture. Korean Circ J 2011;41(7):409–12.

73. Zimarino M, Prati F, Stabile E, et al. Optical coherence tomography accurately identifies intermediate atherosclerotic lesions–an in vivo evaluation in the rabbit carotid artery. Atherosclerosis 2007;193(1):94–101.

74. van Werkum JW, Heestermans AA, Zomer AC, et al. Predictors of coronary stent thrombosis: the Dutch Stent Thrombosis Registry. J Am Coll Cardiol 2009;53(16):1399–409.

75. Nakamura S, Colombo A, Gaglione A, et al. Intracoronary ultrasound observations during stent implantation. Circulation 1994;89(5):2026–34.

76. Zhang Y, Farooq V, Garcia-Garcia HM, et al. Comparison of intravascular ultrasound versus angiography-guided drug-eluting stent implantation: a meta-analysis of one randomised trial and ten observational studies involving 19,619 patients. EuroIntervention 2012;8:855–65.

77. Mattesini A, Pighi M, Konstantinidis N, et al. Optical coherence tomography in bioabsorbable stents: mechanism of vascular response and guidance of stent implantation. Minerva Cardioangiol 2014;62(1):71–82.

78. Mattesini A, Secco GG, Dall'Ara G, et al. ABSORB biodegradable stents versus second-generation metal stents: a comparison study of 100 complex lesions treated under OCT guidance. JACC Cardiovasc Interv 2014;7(7):741–50.

Optical Coherence Tomography in the Diagnosis and Management of Spontaneous Coronary Artery Dissection

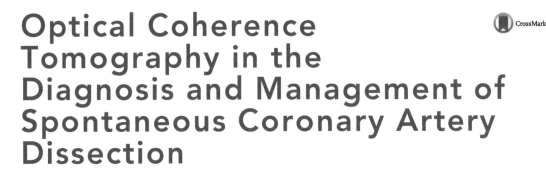

Christopher Franco, MD, PhD, Lim Eng, MD, Jacqueline Saw, MD, FRCPC*

KEYWORDS

• Spontaneous coronary artery dissection • Optical coherence tomography • Intravascular ultrasound • Intracoronary imaging

---

KEY POINTS

• Spontaneous coronary artery dissection (SCAD) is an infrequent condition that has been underdiagnosed and misdiagnosed.
• Use of intracoronary imaging with intravascular ultrasound (IVUS) or optical coherence tomography (OCT) enables the accurate diagnosis of this challenging condition.
• Diagnostic and management algorithms have been proposed to improve the diagnosis and therapeutic stratification of this condition.
• OCT has better spatial resolution than does IVUS and is instrumental in the diagnosis of SCAD cases where angiographic findings are ambiguous for confirming SCAD.
• Understanding the role and appropriate use of this technology is expected to improve the diagnosis of SCAD, and also improve outcomes with percutaneous intervention, when clinically indicated.

SPONTANEOUS CORONARY ARTERY DISSECTION

Epidemiology

Spontaneous coronary artery dissection (SCAD) is a clinically challenging entity that is an important cause of acute myocardial ischemia/infarction and sudden cardiac death in women.[1] The first case of SCAD was described in 1931 on autopsy of a 41-year-old woman presenting with sudden cardiac death and without classic risk factors for atherosclerotic disease. The first angiographic report of SCAD was in 1973 by Forker and colleagues[2] describing the angiographic appearance of extraluminal dye. Since then, fewer than 1000 cases of SCAD have been noted in the medical literature. Retrospective registries have reported SCAD in 0.07% to 1.1% of all coronary angiograms.[3–6] Previous reports have alluded to the rare observation of SCAD as a causative element in acute coronary syndrome (ACS) and sudden cardiac death, accounting for 0.1% to 4% and 0.4%, respectively.[5,7] In a series

---

Disclosures: Dr Saw has received unrestricted research grant supports (from the Canadian Institutes of Health Research, University of British Columbia Division of Cardiology, AstraZeneca, Abbott Vascular, St Jude Medical, Boston Scientific, and Servier), speaker honoraria (AstraZeneca, St Jude Medical, Boston Scientific, Bayer and Sunovion), consultancy and advisory board honoraria (AstraZeneca, St Jude Medical, Boston Scientific, and Abbott Vascular), and proctorship honoraria (St Jude Medical and Boston Scientific). Other authors have no disclosure.
Division of Cardiology, Vancouver General Hospital, University of British Columbia, 2775 Laurel Street, Level 9, Vancouver, BC V5Z1M9, Canada
* Corresponding author.
E-mail address: jsaw@mail.ubc.ca

Intervent Cardiol Clin 4 (2015) 309–320
http://dx.doi.org/10.1016/j.iccl.2015.02.007

by Vanzetto and colleagues,[3] the prevalence was higher among women age younger than 50, where it accounted for 8.7% of troponin-positive ACS. We recently reported a retrospective series in which 24% of women younger than age 50 who were undergoing coronary angiography had angiographically detectable SCAD.[1,8] Taken together, these data suggest that SCAD is much more prevalent than previously considered; however, at present, the true population-based incidence of SCAD remains unknown.

There are several reasons why the incidence of SCAD has been underestimated in the medical literature. The association of SCAD with cardiac arrest may identify a cohort of patients who die before presentation to hospital. Second, many cases of SCAD may have been mistakenly identified as atherosclerotic coronary dissection, which is a mechanically distinct variant from non-atherosclerotic SCAD. Finally, given the often subtle clinical and angiographic presentation, it remains possible that many cases of SCAD have been misdiagnosed as mild atherosclerotic disease or missed altogether.

More recently, through meticulous angiographic review, we and others have described larger cohorts of patients with SCAD and identified SCAD as a far more prevalent cause of ACS in young women.[9–11] In a retrospective single-center cohort study from the Mayo clinic,[10] 87 angiographically confirmed cases of SCAD were identified. Among those with angiographically confirmed SCAD, 82% were female and the mean age was 43 years. The initial clinical presentation was ST-elevation myocardial infarction in 49% of cases. SCAD recurred in 17% with a 10-year recurrence rate of 29%, underscoring the need for close follow-up. In the Madrid cohort,[9] a prospective series of 45 patients with SCAD treated conservatively were followed for more than 6 years. Again, most were young (<50 years old) women presenting with acute myocardial infarction. The predominant angiographic appearance of SCAD in this series was a long diffuse narrowing (type 2 angiographic SCAD, discussed later) rather than presenting as an intimal flap or vessel wall stain. In those cases with angiographic follow-up, more than 50% of SCAD lesions had resolved with conservative therapy, underscoring the natural history of this disease and providing a clear rationale for conservative management.

We recently reported the largest cohort of prospectively and retrospectively identified patients with SCAD (N = 168).[11] In this cohort, 92% of patients were female (62% of whom were post-menopausal) and the mean age was 52. The dominant angiographic appearance of SCAD was again that of a smooth diffuse narrowing (type 2 angiographic SCAD), observed in 67% of cases. We examined the prevalence of potential predisposing conditions and demonstrated evidence of fibromuscular dysplasia (FMD) in 72%. Spontaneous angiographic "healing" of SCAD was observed in all 79 cases with angiographic follow-up, supporting the use of a conservative management strategy in most patients. Taken together, these more recent data identify SCAD as a clinically important cause of ACS in women, and should be considered in the differential diagnosis.

Pathogenesis

SCAD is defined as a nontraumatic and noniatrogenic separation of the coronary arterial wall by intramural hemorrhage and the resultant creation of a false lumen. The dissection plane can occur at the intimal-medial or medial-adventitial interface and need not have an intimal dissection flap.[12] The resulting intramural hematoma (IMH) can occlude or compromise the true vessel lumen leading to myocardial ischemia and infarction.

There are two proposed mechanisms of SCAD (Fig. 1). The first includes initiation of medial dissection and hemorrhage by an intimal tear and creation of a false lumen. The second involves the spontaneous development of an IMH potentially caused by disruption of the intra-arterial vasa vasorum.[13]

The cause of SCAD is multifactorial with contribution of a predisposing arteriopathy (resulting in vulnerable vessel wall segments) and precipitating stressor events. Predisposing arteriopathies can be broadly classified as atherosclerotic SCAD and non-atherosclerotic SCAD (NA-SCAD).[11] Disruption of the atherosclerotic intima can lead to SCAD; however, these dissections tend to be limited in extent by medial atrophy and scarring.[14] Predisposing arteriopathies in NA-SCAD include peripartum (likely a culmination of hormonal exposure and hemodynamic changes during pregnancy), multiple previous pregnancies,[15] connective tissue disorders (eg, Marfan syndrome, Loeys-Dietz syndrome, Ehlers-Danlos syndrome type 4, cystic medial necrosis, α_1-antitrypsin deficiency, and polycystic kidney disease), systemic inflammatory conditions (eg, systemic lupus erythematosus, Crohn disease, ulcerative colitis, polyarteritis nodosa, sarcoidosis, Churg-Strauss syndrome, Wegener granulomatosis, rheumatoid arthritis, Kawasaki, giant cell arteritis, and celiac disease), coronary spasm, or idiopathic.[11]

The predominance of female sex in the SCAD population seems to support a mechanistic role

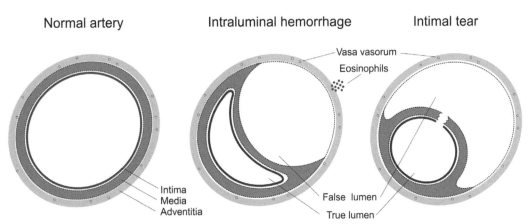

Fig. 1. Schematic illustration of proposed SCAD mechanisms. (*From* Saw J. Spontaneous coronary artery dissection. Can J Cardiol 2013;29:1027–33; with permission.)

for hormonal status in SCAD pathogenesis and earlier reports of SCAD proposed an association with pregnancy and oral contraceptive use.[16,17] Although recent series have challenged this notion, estrogen level and pregnancy status remain important risk factors for SCAD; however, their exact contribution to the pathogenesis of SCAD remains unclear.[11,18]

Precipitating stress events increase shear forces locally and may precipitate SCAD in vulnerable vessel segments. Precipitating events identified in SCAD have included intense exercise (isometric or aerobic), intense emotional stress, labor and delivery, intense Valsalva-type activities (eg, retching, vomiting, bowel movement, and coughing), sympathomimetic drugs (eg, cocaine, amphetamines, and methamphetamines), and intense hormonal therapy (eg, β-human chorionic gonadotropin injections). In our series, more than half of patients who presented with SCAD reported a precipitating stressor.[11]

The relative frequency of predisposing and precipitating factors in the pathogenesis remains an area of active investigation. We recently reported a large SCAD cohort and identified several predisposing arteriopathies, with the most prevalent being FMD (72%), idiopathic (20.1%), and hormonal therapy (10.7%).[11]

Fibromuscular Dysplasia

FMD is a segmental nonatherosclerotic, noninflammatory, vasculopathy of the small to medium sized arteries that can affect all layers of the vessel wall. Historically, FMD was classified histologically into intimal fibroplasia, medial fibroplasia (correlating with the angiographic string-of-beads appearance), medial hyperplasia, perimedial fibroplasia, and adventitial fibroplasia.[19,20] Case reports have demonstrated severe disorganization of the ultrastructure of

the arterial wall with alternating areas of smooth muscle cells hyperplasia and adventitial collagen deposition with loss of the anatomic boundaries of the elastic lamellae, all contributing to severe luminal obstruction. The first case of coronary FMD associated with SCAD was reported in 1987 by autopsy.[19] Multiple case reports, including our own, have since implicated coronary FMD as a central predisposing arteriopathy in the pathogenesis of SCAD.[11,19,21–27] Intracoronary imaging with intravascular ultrasound (IVUS) and optical coherence tomography (OCT) can document areas of bright, echogenic/reflective collagen interspersed with areas of cellular hyperplasia similar to the histologic descriptions of FMD.[24]

Angiographically, coronary FMD may appear with the classical description of medial fibroplasia with string-of-beads appearance, but this is relatively infrequent.[28] More commonly, coronary FMD may appear normal angiographically because small arterioles may be involved, with suspected microvascular dysfunction. Other appearances on coronary angiography include diffuse stenosis, tubular stenosis, and ectasia. In patients presenting with overlying SCAD on pre-existing FMD, the characteristic acute angiographic appearance of SCAD may be observed (discussed later). This appearance normalizes with resorption of the IMH that occurs with healing of the dissection.

The diagnosis of coronary FMD remains challenging and much of the data supporting an association between FMD and SCAD have emerged from the incidental detection of renal and iliofemoral FMD observed during routine coronary angiography. Our group described the first series of SCAD with incidental FMD.[26,29] Furthermore, in our initial cohort of 50 patients with SCAD, 86% had concomitant renal, iliofemoral, or cerebrovascular FMD.[8] These findings were supported by previous reports[10] noting an association with iliofemoral FMD in cases of SCAD. In our more recent, larger series of 168 patients with SCAD, we detected FMD in 72% of cases.[11] Given this frequent association, we suspect that previous cases of idiopathic SCAD may have had underlying undiagnosed FMD.

Angiographic Features of Spontaneous Coronary Artery Dissection: the Saw Angiographic Spontaneous Coronary Artery Dissection Classification

The two-dimensional luminogram offered by traditional angiography is indispensible for the rapid evaluation of patients with acute myocardial ischemia. However, the main limitation of angiography is its inability to visualize the layers of the coronary vessel wall. The diagnosis of SCAD relies on often subtle angiographic features, and careful attention to vessel opacification and stenosis characterization are critical to help differentiate IMH from other causes of coronary stenosis. The administration of intra-arterial vasodilators is important to rule out the contribution of arterial spasm to subtle narrowings. Because patients with SCAD often have generalized coronary arterial fragility, a cautious and meticulous approach to performing coronary angiography is advised; for example, avoiding catheter-dampening, deep catheter engagements, and strong injections of contrast.

Early identification of SCAD is paramount in the management of patients presenting with ACS, because the therapeutic strategy for SCAD differs significantly from the treatment of atherosclerotic stenosis. Coronary angiography provides two-dimensional assessment of coronary anatomy and the grade of coronary flow. It remains the mainstay of investigation in patients with suspected SCAD. Pathognomonic angiographic appearances may include multiple radiolucent lines, false lumen, contrast staining, and late contrast clearing, all of which are consistent with intimal tear.

Saw proposed three distinctive angiographic patterns to improve the diagnostic accuracy of SCAD.[30] Type 1 (evident arterial wall stain) has the characteristically described angiographic appearance and is easily detected on coronary angiography (Fig. 2). Type 2 (diffuse stenosis of varying severity) is the most common form of SCAD accounting for 67% of cases.[11] It involves predominantly the mid to distal coronary segments with subtle but abrupt change in

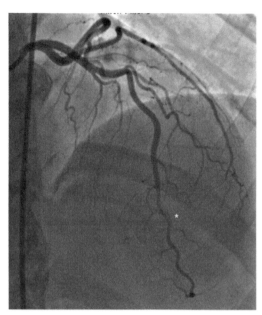

Fig. 2. Type 1 angiographic SCAD (according to angiographic classification by Saw criteria) of the distal left anterior descending with contrast arterial wall stain (*asterisk*).

vessel caliber. Some cases may appear diffuse (typically >20 mm) and usually with smooth narrowing (Fig. 3). Type 3 (mimic atherosclerosis) cannot be distinguished from atherosclerotic stenosis on coronary angiography and is virtually impossible to diagnose without the adjunctive use of intracoronary imaging (Fig. 4). It may have suggestive features, such as long length (11–20 mm), a hazy or linear stenosis, and an absence of atherosclerotic changes in the other coronary arteries.[30]

Intracoronary Imaging of Spontaneous Coronary Artery Dissection

By virtue of its inability to visualize the coronary arterial wall, traditional angiography has limited diagnostic accuracy in SCAD.[5,6] Intracoronary imaging with tomographic techniques including IVUS[13] and OCT[31] can provide a direct assessment of the ultrastructure of the arterial wall and its intimal contents. IVUS has a spatial resolution of 150 μm with deeper tissue penetration, and although it cannot identify intimal tears well, it can readily identify IMH as a homogenous collection behind an intimal-medial membrane.[32] OCT generates three-dimensional images from optical scattering within tissue and has a spatial resolution of 10 to 15 μm.[33,34] On OCT imaging, fibrous tissue and collagen appear bright (high reflectivity),

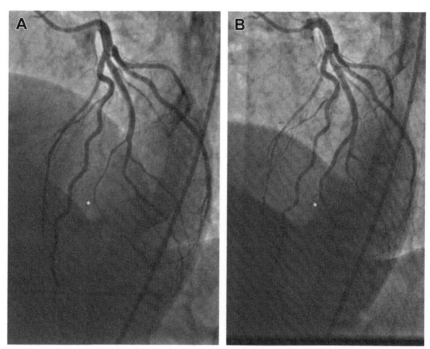

Fig. 3. Type 2 angiographic SCAD (Saw criteria). (*A*) Mid to distal segment of a large diagonal branch (*asterisk*). (*B*) Spontaneous angiographic healing of this diagonal branch on repeat angiogram 1 year later (*asterisk*).

whereas areas of smooth muscle hyperplasia or hematoma appear dark (low reflectivity).[24,35] OCT has significant advantages over IVUS in the diagnosis of SCAD because of its superior spatial resolution, its ability to differentiate clearly between IMH and lipid-rich or calcified atheroma,[31,35,36] and its ability to identify intimal tears or entry sites of dissection.

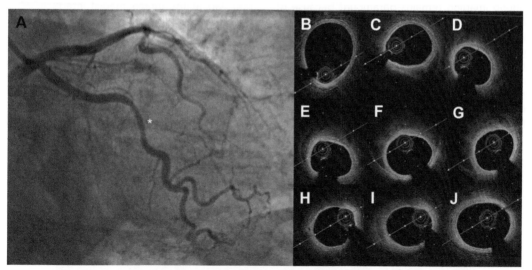

Fig. 4. Type 3 angiographic SCAD (Saw criteria) with (*A*) angiogram showing moderate 60% stenosis of the mid circumflex artery (*asterisk*). (*B–J*) OCT showing IMH. (*B*) Proximal normal segment. (*C*) IMH from 3 to 9 o'clock. (*D*) IMH from 10 to 4 o'clock with thickened intimal-medial membrane separating true from false lumen, but the full depth of IMH was not visualized. (*E*) Crescent-shaped false lumen filled with IMH from 7 to 4 o'clock. (*F*) Crescent-shaped false lumen with IMH of heterogeneous reflexivity caused by heterogeneity of coagulated blood in false lumen, with full extent of IMH well visualized from 7 to 12 o'clock. (*G*) IMH from 7 to 2 o'clock with heterogeneous reflexivity. (*H*) IMH from 8 to 1 o'clock. (*I*) Edge of the dissected artery with thin crescent-shaped IMH from 8 to 1 o'clock. (*J*) Segment distal to dissection showing thickened and fibrotic intima-media.

ROLE OF OPTICAL COHERENCE TOMOGRAPHY IN THE DIAGNOSIS AND MANAGEMENT OF SPONTANEOUS CORONARY ARTERY DISSECTION

Diagnosis

The development of OCT has revolutionized the diagnosis of patients with SCAD, which has been challenging especially in those who present without type 1 angiographic appearance. OCT uses the principle of reflected light for the generation of intraluminal images. Since its first introduction in 1991,[37] it has gained popularity as a diagnostic tool in various medical specialities including coronary intervention. Near-infrared light of 1250 to 1350 nm wavelength is aimed at a target and subsequently the resulting intensity and echo time delay from the reflected light are measured by interferometer for image acquisition. It produces unprecedentedly superior image resolution (axial resolution of 10 μm and lateral resolution of 20 μm) allowing comprehensive visualization and assessment of coronary anatomy and pathology.

There are two types of OCT systems: time domain and frequency domain. Frequency domain OCT system is capable of measuring all echoes of light from different depths simultaneously instead of sequentially as of its earlier counterpart, time domain OCT system, enhancing the sensitivity and speed of acquisition.[38] Nevertheless, creating a blood-free field during imaging remains paramount because of the inability of OCT to image through blood; this may significantly jeopardize the quality of generated images if blood is not cleared from the lumen sufficiently. To achieve this, two techniques were described. The occlusive technique that used a proximal occlusion balloon while flushing a crystalloid solution had fallen out of favor because of concerns of potential coronary ischemia. Nonocclusive flushing of the guide with contrast is now the routine technique, using a frequency domain OCT short monorail catheter (Dragonfly Duo; St Jude Medical, St. Paul, MN) on a coronary guidewire. It allows rapid automated pullback of 18 to 36 mm/s at up to 75 mm in length. Injection of contrast boluses displaces blood from the imaging plane before image acquisition.[39] Optimal and cautious engagement of guiding catheter is crucial to guarantee adequate flushing of blood from the imaging plane during acquisition.

The limitations of coronary angiography in diagnosing SCAD were alluded to previously. Alfonso and colleagues[31] reported that only 3 out of 11 patients with confirmed SCAD on OCT had an intimal flap on coronary angiography. This finding was corroborated by a more contemporary case series that demonstrated that less than 30% of patients with SCAD presented with a classical, type 1 angiographic appearances.[11] This in large part explains the underdiagnosis of SCAD in the past, compounded by the lack of appropriate intracoronary imaging and knowledge of this clinical entity at the time. Moreover, type 2 and 3 SCADs are easily missed using conventional angiography.

OCT has proved to be an invaluable imaging modality in guiding the diagnosis of patients with suspected SCAD.[31,35,40,41] It facilitates the visualization of IMH, double lumen, and dissection flap at the intimal-medial interface, which are readily defined on OCT (Fig. 5). Alfonso and colleagues[31] reported the largest prospective series of SCAD with OCT. In this report, 17 cases with features suspicious for SCAD on traditional angiography were assessed by OCT, of which SCAD was confirmed in 11. Among those cases with confirmed SCAD, 82% were female, and the mean age was 48 years. The

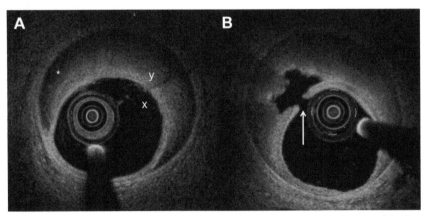

Fig. 5. OCT images showing (A) IMH (*asterisk*) and double-lumen (x = true lumen, and y = false lumen), and (B) intimal tear (*arrow*).

characteristic double lumen was seen in all cases; however, only 3 of 11 had a distinct intimal flap or entry point, with the remainder showing IMH only, without intimal flap. All patients had associated thrombus in either true or false lumens. The intimal-medial membranes in these patients were relatively thick (348 ± 84 μm) with the thinnest at the edges of the intimal tear.[31] OCT also allows for detailed assessment and identification of the precise origin of intimal disruption, the length of affected vessel, thickness and distribution of dissection flap, magnitude of luminal compromise, side-branch involvement, and associated thrombus formation. All this information is valuable when planning coronary intervention.

Nevertheless, because most SCAD cases may be managed conservatively without percutaneous coronary intervention (PCI), the dominant role of OCT in this condition is simply to make the diagnosis of SCAD. For this purpose, the OCT catheter need not be placed across the full length of the dissection. In our practice, the OCT catheter imaging tip is placed at the beginning of the suspected dissected segment, and a "live-view" image is then assessed to seek for IMH. If the catheter is not occlusive, we then perform contrast injection to activate the imaging pull-back.

In our proposed diagnostic algorithm (Fig. 6), early coronary angiography should be offered to all patients with suspected SCAD. Type 1 SCAD is readily identified by angiography alone. In the absence of this pathognomonic angiographic appearance, OCT or IVUS is recommended for further assessment. In patients who display type 2 appearance, intracoronary nitroglycerine should be administered to eliminate the possibility of coronary spasm. If the type 2 appearance persists, intracoronary imaging should be performed if the diagnosis is uncertain, or alternatively, coronary angiography can be repeated 4 to 6 weeks later to confirm the diagnosis when angiographic healing occurs. Type 3 appearances should always be investigated with intracoronary imaging because it is practically indistinct to atherosclerosis angiographically.[30]

Optical coherence tomography guidance for percutaneous coronary intervention

PCI in patients with SCAD is technically demanding and challenging. Wiring the true lumen poses the risk of propagation of the dissection plane, whereas deploying a coronary stent within the false lumen is potentially disastrous. In these circumstances, OCT is essential in providing unique anatomic and morphologic insights that would otherwise be missed using conventional angiography. Under direct visualization, OCT confirms the positioning of the coronary guidewire in the true lumen, the accurate

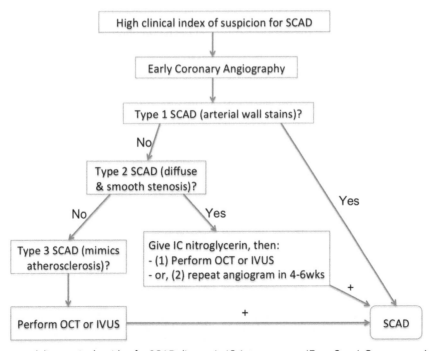

Fig. 6. Suggested diagnostic algorithm for SCAD diagnosis. IC, intracoronary. (*From* Saw J. Coronary angiogram classification of spontaneous coronary artery dissection. Catheter Cardiovasc Interv 2014;84(7):1115–22; with permission.)

localization of the intimal disruption site, and the full extent of IMH involved, thereby facilitating stent sizing and deployment. Adequate apposition of deployed stent struts is readily assessed using OCT (Fig. 7A), and this is important to avoid late stent thrombosis related to malapposition. This risk can be increased with acquired malapposition following resorption of the IMH with dissection healing (see Fig. 7B).

The main limitation encountered when using OCT is the necessity to establish a blood-free environment during imaging. Dissected intimal flaps are generally fragile and at risk of further extension. There are concerns that contrast flushes of even a minimal amount and force may generate considerable hydraulic pressure and propagate axial dissection, thereby compromising coronary flow distally. However, this risk seems theoretic and we have not encountered complications related to hydraulic dissection in our small series of SCAD intracoronary imaging.[42] Another limitation of OCT is the poor depth of tissue penetration (1–2.5 mm), which can result in failure to depict the entire thickness of the dissected plane and IMH. Significant attenuation caused by red thrombus in the false lumen may in turn degrade the quality of the generated images. However, these limitations should not significantly limit the use of OCT during PCI, which should predominantly entail true lumen access, dissection length assessment, and stent strut apposition.

Spontaneous coronary artery dissection diagnosis with intravascular ultrasound

IVUS is an alternative form of intracoronary imaging frequently used in clinical practice. It relies on the emission and backscattering of ultrasonic waves that are converted to electrical signals to generate images. However, the resolution of IVUS is inferior to OCT (axial resolution, 150 μm). Maehara and colleagues[43] first described the effectiveness of IVUS in diagnosing cases of SCAD without characteristic angiographic features. In this small cases series, IVUS identified five patients who had medial dissection related to IMH in the absence of a concomitant intimal tear. Similarly, Arnold and colleagues[32] validated the clinical application of IVUS in the diagnosis of four patients with SCAD. Overall, IVUS is useful to confirm the presence of IMH and a double lumen, identify the true lumen, and identify the severity of luminal compression; however, when compared with OCT, IVUS is inferior in indentifying intimal tears.

Although there are complimentary roles for OCT and IVUS in SCAD imaging, the costs of both imaging modalities preclude their simultaneous use in most laboratories. Despite its superior imaging resolution, OCT is insufficient in tissue penetration, preventing detailed assessment of the full thickness of dissection plane involved. Most of the outer border of vessel wall is poorly visualized. However, IVUS with its higher tissue penetration strength (10 mm) enables the evaluation of the external elastic lamina and the entire extent of dissected segments, even in patients with large-caliber coronary vessels or intraluminal red thrombus.[40] Paulo and colleagues[44] prospectively examined the combined use of OCT and IVUS in the assessment of patients with SCAD. OCT was superior to IVUS in the recognition of intimal ruptures and intraluminal thrombi. The presence of a false lumen and IMH was well elucidated by OCT, but their full extent could not be determined because of shadowing interference and inadequate penetration. This was easily overcome by concomitant use of

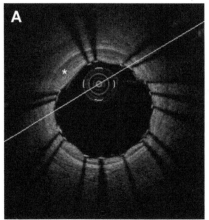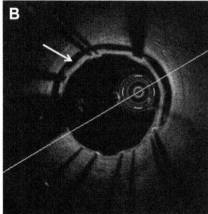

Fig. 7. OCT images showing (A) stent strut apposition during acute stent procedure (*asterisk*), and (B) gaps behind the stent struts at intermediate 2-week follow-up caused by resorption of intramural hematoma (*arrow*).

IVUS, which provided complete vessel visualization with the assessment of significantly longer diseased segment and larger false lumen areas. Thrombus with heterogeneous appearance in the false lumen is readily illustrated on IVUS.[45] Poon and colleagues[45] also illustrated the successful use of the combination of IVUS and OCT in guiding PCI.

Management of Spontaneous Coronary Artery Dissection

The optimal management strategy and medical therapy for SCAD is unknown and is largely empirical given the absence of randomized studies. Apart from anecdotal reports regarding clinical outcomes, there is little evidence-based guidance on criteria for revascularization or methods to perform such revascularization. A high index of clinical suspicion in an appropriate context is crucial and may pre-empt the use of unnecessary and potential harmful therapies. Serial angiographic reports have supported the notion that the natural history of SCAD involves complete healing in patients managed without intervention, and therefore a conservative management strategy is appropriate in most cases.[9–11] Fig. 8 illustrates a simple

management algorithm regarding the need for revascularization according to the clinical status of patients presenting with SCAD.[11] Revascularization for SCAD should be considered in patients with active myocardial ischemia or hemodynamic instability. PCI should be considered in patients with localized proximal dissections in large vessels associated with ongoing ischemia or reduced TIMI flow. Coronary artery bypass graft should be reserved for patients with left main or multivessel proximal large-vessel dissection, especially in the setting of hemodynamic compromise. However, graft patency failure after the resolution of the IMH and restoration of native coronary flow has been reported, presumably caused by competitive flow in the native arteries.[10,11]

With regards to medical management, we have previously published a review of the available literature.[1] We advocate routine long-term therapy with aspirin and a β-blocker following SCAD presentation, if tolerated. It is hoped that the SAFER-SCAD study (NCT02008786), a small, prospective randomized trial to evaluate the use of statin and angiotensin-converting enzyme inhibitor in the setting of SCAD, will provide some guidance on the management of this condition.

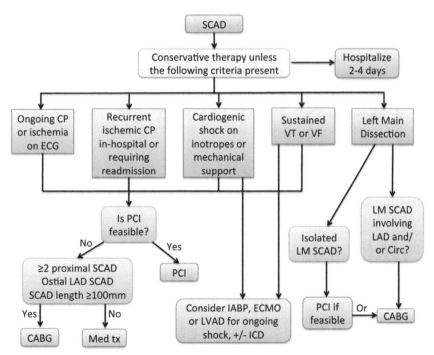

Fig. 8. Recommended management algorithm. CABG, coronary artery bypass graft; CP, chest pain; ECG, electrocardiogram; ECMO, extracorporeal membrane oxygenation; IABP, intraaortic balloon pump; ICD, implantable cardiac defibrillator; LAD, left anterior descending; LM, left main; LVAD, left-ventricular assist device; tx, treatment; VT, ventricular tachycardia. (*From* Saw J, Aymong E, Sedlak T, et al. Spontaneous coronary artery dissection: association with predisposing arteriopathies and precipitating stressors and cardiovascular outcomes. Circ Cardiovasc Interv 2014;7:645–55; with permission.)

PCI in SCAD is associated with significant technical difficulties attributed to the fragility of the vessel wall. Technical difficulties might include guidewire placement in the true lumen, dissection in small-caliber distal vessels, risk of dissection propagation, and side branch occlusion. Care must be taken to avoid stent or vessel overdilation, which may lead to propagation of the dissection or perforation.[27] In addition, SCAD segments frequently require long stent length, thereby increasing the risk of restenosis. Direct stenting may be preferable to predilation when possible, and the stent placement can be guided by OCT. To mitigate propagation of the dissection, some groups[9,46] have proposed OCT-guided stent deployment at the proximal and distal ends of the dissection before stenting the middle segment. Finally, the temporal resolution of IMH in previously stented segments may increase the risk of late stent malapposition and subsequent stent thrombosis.[18] In all cases, avoiding overstenting and "full metal jacket" is important. The use of bioabsorbable scaffolds in treating SCAD is theoretically appealing, because it allows local "sealing" of the dissection entry site and addresses the problem of late stent malapposition after resorption of the residual IMH.

Multiple reports have identified generally poor technical results with PCI for SCAD. In our recent cohort of 168 patients, 33 underwent PCI, which was unsuccessful in 12 cases (36%). Of those cases with successful or partially successful PCI, 57% had extension of dissection, and 6%, 24%, and 12% had subsequent stent thrombosis, restenosis, or required coronary artery bypass graft, respectively. Overall the number of PCIs with a durable, successful result was a meager 30%.[11] These findings are supported by a previous report that demonstrated a PCI failure rate of 35% in SCAD.[8,10] The radial approach may be associated with increased risk of iatrogenic dissections in patients with SCAD, with 3 of 41 radial angiograms resulting in iatrogenic dissection secondary to deep intubation of the left main coronary ostium. By contrast, no dissections were noted in the patients with femoral access.[11] Clearly, meticulous angiographic techniques are crucial in this complex population and with particular attention to avoid deep intubation and pressure damping.

Future Directions

The addition of OCT to the interventional cardiologists' armamentarium has fundamentally changed the ability to diagnose and manage SCAD. OCT continues to provide novel insight into this important disease through the identification of new cases, unparalleled visualization of its pathogenesis, and the ability to evaluate the local effect of novel therapies. Micro-OCT, a three-dimensional imaging technique with unprecedented 1- to 2-μm spatial resolution, has the promise to provide subcellular insight into the in vivo vascular biology of vulnerable vessel segments, potentially before their dissection.[47] For instance, in patients with coexisting FMD, it will be remarkable to evaluate the coronary artery for histologic FMD changes adjacent to dissected segments to better understand the mechanism predisposing to SCAD. Despite these advances, a major hurdle in this field remains the paucity of randomized data and evidence-based guidelines to direct the care of this complex patient population. Further prospective studies defining the optimal medical therapy and long-term outcomes are needed.

SUMMARY

In summary, SCAD is an infrequent condition that has been underdiagnosed and misdiagnosed. The use of intracoronary imaging with IVUS or OCT enables the accurate diagnosis of this challenging condition. Diagnostic and management algorithms have been proposed to improve the diagnosis and therapeutic stratification of this condition. OCT has superior spatial resolution than IVUS, and is instrumental in the diagnosis of SCAD cases where angiographic findings are ambiguous for confirming SCAD. Understanding the role and appropriate and careful use of this technology is expected to improve the diagnosis of SCAD, and also improve outcomes with PCI, when clinically indicated.

REFERENCES

1. Saw J. Spontaneous coronary artery dissection. Can J Cardiol 2013;29:1027–33.
2. Forker AD, Rosenlof RC, Weaver WF, et al. Primary dissecting aneurysm of the right coronary artery with survival. Chest 1973;64:656–8.
3. Vanzetto G, Berger-Coz E, Barone-Rochette G, et al. Prevalence, therapeutic management and medium-term prognosis of spontaneous coronary artery dissection: results from a database of 11,605 patients. Eur J Cardiothorac Surg 2009;35:250–4.
4. Shamloo BK, Chintala RS, Nasur A, et al. Spontaneous coronary artery dissection: aggressive vs. conservative therapy. J Invasive Cardiol 2010;22:222.
5. Mortensen KH, Thuesen L, Kristensen IB. Spontaneous coronary artery dissection: a Western Denmark Heart Registry study. Catheter Cardiovasc Interv 2009;74:710–7.

6. Vrints C. Spontaneous coronary artery dissection. Heart 2010;96:801–8.

7. Hill SF, Sheppard MN. Non-atherosclerotic coronary artery disease associated with sudden cardiac death. Heart 2010;96:1119–25.

8. Saw J, Ricci D, Starovoytov A, et al. Spontaneous coronary artery dissection: prevalence of predisposing conditions including fibromuscular dysplasia in a tertiary center cohort. JACC Cardiovasc Interv 2013;6:44–52.

9. Alfonso F, Paulo M, Lennie V, et al. Spontaneous coronary artery dissection: long-term follow-up of a large series of patients prospectively managed with a "conservative" therapeutic strategy. JACC Cardiovasc Interv 2012;5:1062–70.

10. Tweet MS, Hayes SN, Pitta SR, et al. Clinical features, management, and prognosis of spontaneous coronary artery dissection. Circulation 2012;126:579–88.

11. Saw J, Aymong E, Sedlak T, et al. Spontaneous coronary artery dissection: association with predisposing arteriopathies and precipitating stressors and cardiovascular outcomes. Circ Cardiovasc Interv 2014;7:645–55.

12. Reynolds H. Mechanisms of myocardial infarction without obstructive coronary artery disease. Trends Cardiovasc Med 2014;24:170–6.

13. Maehara A, Mintz GS, Ahmed JM, et al. An intravascular ultrasound classification of angiographic coronary artery aneurysms. Am J Cardiol 2001;88:365–70.

14. Isner JM, Donaldson RF, Fortin AH, et al. Attenuation of the media of coronary arteries in advanced atherosclerosis. Am J Cardiol 1986;58:937–9.

15. Vijayaraghavan R, Verma S, Gupta N, et al. Clinician update: pregnancy-related spontaneous coronary artery dissection. Circulation 2014;130(21):1915–20.

16. Koul AK, Hollander G, Moskovits N. Coronary artery dissection during pregnancy and the postpartum period: two case reports and review of literature. Catheter Cardiovasc Interv 2001;52:88–94.

17. Giacoppo D, Capodanno D, Dangas G, et al. Spontaneous coronary artery dissection. Int J Cardiol 2014;175:8–20.

18. Alfonso F, Bastante T, Rivero F, et al. Spontaneous coronary artery dissection. Circ J 2014;78:2099–110.

19. Lie JT, Berg KK. Isolated fibromuscular dysplasia of the coronary arteries with spontaneous dissection and myocardial infarction. Hum Pathol 1987;18:654–6.

20. Harrison EG Jr, McCormack LJ. Pathologic classification of renal arterial disease in renovascular hypertension. Mayo Clin Proc 1971;46(3):161–7.

21. Brodsky SV, Ramaswamy G, Chander P, et al. Ruptured cerebral aneurysm and acute coronary artery dissection in the setting of multivascular fibromuscular dysplasia a case report. Angiology 2008;58:764.

22. Mather PJ, Hansen CL, Goldman B. Postpartum multivessel coronary dissection. J Heart Lung Transplant 1993;13(3):533–7.

23. Saw J, Aymong E, Mancini G, et al. Nonatherosclerotic coronary artery disease in young women. Can J Cardiol 2014;30:814–9.

24. Saw J, Poulter R, Fung A. Intracoronary imaging of coronary fibromuscular dysplasia with OCT and IVUS. Catheter Cardiovasc Interv 2013;82:E879–83.

25. Garcia NA, Khan AN, Boppana RC, et al. Spontaneous coronary artery dissection: a case series and literature review. J Community Hosp Intern Med Perspect 2014;4:1–5.

26. Pate GE, Lowe R, Buller CE. Fibromuscular dysplasia of the coronary and renal arteries? Catheter Cardiovasc Interv 2005;64:138–45.

27. Poulter R, Ricci D, Saw J. Perforation during stenting of a coronary artery with morphologic changes of fibromuscular dysplasia: an unrecognized risk with percutaneous intervention. Can J Cardiol 2013;29:519.e1–3.

28. Michelis K, Olin J, Kadian-Dodov D, et al. Coronary artery manifestations of fibromuscular dysplasia. J Am Coll Cardiol 2014;64:1033–46.

29. Saw J, Poulter R, Fung A, et al. Spontaneous coronary artery dissection in patients with fibromuscular dysplasia: a case series. Circ Cardiovasc Interv 2012;5:134–7.

30. Saw J. Coronary angiogram classification of spontaneous coronary artery dissection. Catheter Cardiovasc Interv 2014;84(7):1115–22.

31. Alfonso F, Paulo M, Gonzalo N, et al. Diagnosis of spontaneous coronary artery dissection by optical coherence tomography. J Am Coll Cardiol 2012;59:1073–9.

32. Arnold JR, West NE, van Gaal WJ, et al. The role of intravascular ultrasound in the management of spontaneous coronary artery dissection. Cardiovasc Ultrasound 2008;6:24.

33. Abtahian F, Jang IK. Optical coherence tomography: basics, current application and future potential. Curr Opin Pharmacol 2012;12:583–91.

34. Alfonso F, Canales E, Aleong G. Spontaneous coronary artery dissection: diagnosis by optical coherence tomography. Eur Heart J 2009;30:385.

35. Lim C, Banning A, Channon K. Optical coherence tomography in the diagnosis and treatment of spontaneous coronary artery dissection. J Invasive Cardiol 2010;22:559–60.

36. Prati F, Regar E, Mintz GS, et al. Expert review document on methodology, terminology, and clinical applications of optical coherence tomography. Eur Heart J 2010;31:401–15.

37. Huang D, Swanson EA, Lin CP, et al. Optical coherence tomography. Science 1991;254:1178–81.

38. Lowe HC, Narula J, Fujimoto JG, et al. Intracoronary optical diagnostics current status, limitations, and potential. JACC Cardiovasc Interv 2011;4:1257–70.

39. Prati F, Cera M, Ramazzotti V, et al. Safety and feasibility of a new non-occlusive technique for facilitated intracoronary optical coherence tomography (OCT) acquisition in various clinical and anatomical scenarios. EuroIntervention 2007;3:365–70.

40. Alfonso F, Paulo M, Dutary J. Endovascular imaging of angiographically invisible spontaneous coronary artery dissection. JACC Cardiovasc Interv 2012;5:452–3.

41. Ishibashi K, Kitabata H, Akasaka T. Intracoronary optical coherence tomography assessment of spontaneous coronary artery dissection. Heart 2009;95:818.

42. Saw J, Mancini GBJ, Humphries K, et al. Angiographic appearance of spontaneous coronary artery dissection with intramural hematoma proven on intracoronary imaging. J Am Coll Cardiol 2014;64:B3.

43. Maehara A, Mintz GS, Castagna MT, et al. Intravascular ultrasound assessment of spontaneous coronary artery dissection. Am J Cardiol 2002;89:466–8.

44. Paulo M, Sandoval J, Lennie V, et al. Combined use of OCT and IVUS in spontaneous coronary artery dissection. JACC Cardiovasc Imaging 2013;6:830–2.

45. Poon K, Bell B, Raffel OC, et al. Spontaneous coronary artery dissection: utility of intravascular ultrasound and optical coherence tomography during percutaneous coronary intervention. Circ Cardiovasc Interv 2011;4:e5–7.

46. Walsh SJ, Jokhi PP, Saw J. Successful percutaneous management of coronary dissection and extensive intramural haematoma associated with ST elevation MI. Acute Card Care 2008;10:231–3.

47. Liu L, Gardecki J, Nadkarni S, et al. Imaging the subcellular structure of human coronary atherosclerosis using micro-optical coherence tomography. Nat Med 2011;17:1010–4.

Neointimal Coverage After Drug-Eluting Stent Implantation
Insights from Optical Coherence Tomography

Seung-Yul Lee, MD[a], Myeong-Ki Hong, MD, PhD[b,c,d,*]

KEYWORDS

• Drug-eluting stent • Neointima • Optical coherence tomography

KEY POINTS

- Compared with first-generation drug-eluting stents (DES), second-generation DES are associated with better strut coverage and lower incidence of stent thrombosis, suggesting shorter duration of dual antiplatelet therapy.
- As delayed neointimal healing is commonly observed in large DES malapposition, stent optimization strategy using optical coherence tomography (OCT) may have clinical benefits.
- In the late phase after DES implantation, neoatherosclerosis contributes to progressive neointimal growth and unstable clinical presentation such as acute coronary syndrome or stent thrombosis.
- Besides neoatherosclerosis, various types of neointimal tissue on OCT have been under investigation.

INTRODUCTION

Intravascular ultrasonography has traditionally been considered the gold standard for invasive coronary imaging. Several studies using intravascular ultrasonography have revealed the pathophysiology of coronary artery disease and have led to the improvement of stent therapy. Recently, optical coherence tomography (OCT) has been applied to intravascular imaging.[1]

OCT uses near-infrared light, and has a better resolution (10–20 μm) than intravascular ultrasonography (80–120 μm). This high resolution uniquely enables the visualization of early-phase vascular responses after stent implantation. Compared with intravascular ultrasonography, OCT has better diagnostic accuracy for detecting a small amount of neointima, which has been defined as that occupying less than 30% of stent area.[2] In other report, OCT was able to detect

Funding Sources: This study was supported by a grant from the Korea Healthcare Technology R&D Project, Ministry of Health, Welfare and Family Affairs, Republic of Korea (Nos. A085012 and A102064), and a grant from the Korea Health 21 R&D Project, Ministry of Health and Welfare, Republic of Korea (No. A085136), and the Cardiovascular Research Center, Seoul, Korea.

a Division of Cardiology, Sanbon Hospital, Wonkwang University College of Medicine, 321 Sabbonno, Gunpo, Gyeonggido 435-040, Korea; b Division of Cardiology, Severance Cardiovascular Hospital, Yonsei University College of Medicine, Yonsei University Health System, 250 Seongsanno, Seodaemun-gu, Seoul 120-752, Korea; c Cardiovascular Institute, Yonsei University College of Medicine, 250 Seongsanno, Seodaemun-gu, Seoul 120-752, Korea; d Severance Biomedical Science Institute, Yonsei University College of Medicine, 250 Seongsanno, Seodaemun-gu, Seoul 120-752, Korea

* Corresponding author. Division of Cardiology, Severance Cardiovascular Hospital, Yonsei University College of Medicine, 250 Seongsanno, Seodaemun-gu, Seoul 120-752, Korea.
E-mail address: mkhong61@yuhs.ac

percent neointimal area of less than 14.7%, a level intravascular ultrasonography could not achieve.[3] Recently, frequency-domain OCT technology replaced the time-domain system, which required a proximal occlusion balloon to clear the coronary lumen from blood and acquire images. This procedure was inconvenient and carried a greater risk of myocardial ischemia. However, with the advent of frequency-domain OCT, occlusion of the proximal portion of the lesion of interest is not required, because imaging frames are acquired at much higher rates and therefore allow for faster pullback speeds. This advance has led to shorter procedural times (3.2 ± 0.8 vs 11.2 ± 2.5 minutes, $P<.01$) and a higher acquisition rate of clear images (99.4% vs 80.8%, $P<.01$) than with time-domain OCT.[4] With the improvement of OCT systems, novel findings regarding the pathophysiology of stent therapy have been reported. This review describes recent advances in the understanding of neointimal formation derived from OCT imaging of lesions treated with drug-eluting stents (DES).

DELAYED NEOINTIMAL HEALING OF DRUG-ELUTING STENTS

Neointimal formation after stent implantation consists of 3 phases: (1) inflammation, (2) granulation, and (3) tissue remodeling.[5] Bare-metal stent (BMS) studies demonstrate that immediately after stent deployment, most endothelial cells are disrupted. A thin layer of fibrin clot forms over the area of injury. As endothelial cells regenerate and migrate, smooth muscle cells replace fibrin with granulation tissue, facilitated by various growth factors and cytokines.[5] The granulation tissue matures over several months,

along with the stabilization of extracellular matrix. However, the vascular response to DES implantation differs from the response to BMS. Pathologic studies have demonstrated that arterial healing is delayed within first-generation DES when compared with BMS of similar implant duration.[6] Although the mechanisms of delayed healing are multifactorial, antiproliferative drugs such as sirolimus or paclitaxel are mainly involved. These drugs inhibit not only the proliferation and migration of smooth muscle cells but also regrowth of injured endothelial cells.[7] Thus, persistent fibrin deposition around stent struts or poor endothelialization has been commonly observed in DES.[6,7]

Delayed neointimal healing was significantly associated with stent thrombosis, a fatal complication of DES therapy. In particular, signs of delayed healing were greater in postmortem specimens with thrombosed DES, manifested by an increased fibrin score and less endothelial coverage of stent struts.[8] Thus, the most powerful histologic risk factor for stent thrombosis was a lack of endothelial coverage represented by the ratio of uncovered to total stent struts.[8] OCT allows for exquisite detection of strut coverage, and can therefore be used to indirectly assess neointimal healing (Fig. 1). In vivo OCT studies also suggest that delayed coverage of stent struts is a potential mechanism of late stent thrombosis.[9,10] In a cross-sectional OCT study, uncovered struts and positive remodeling were associated with late stent thrombosis after DES implantation.[9] Another OCT study suggested that a cutoff value of 5.9% of uncovered struts measured at 6 to 18 months after DES implantation could predict major adverse cardiac events, including stent thrombosis.[10]

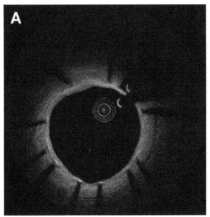 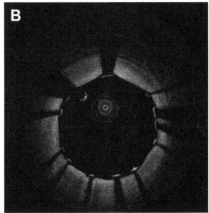

Fig. 1. Covered and uncovered struts detected by optical coherence tomography (OCT). (A) Covered struts. (B) Uncovered struts.

STRUT COVERAGE WITH NEWER-GENERATION DRUG-ELUTING STENTS

Several OCT studies have investigated DES strut coverage at various time intervals of follow-up.[11–16] At 6 months, the sirolimus-eluting stent (SES; Cypher, Cordis, Miami, FL, USA) showed 11% of uncovered struts,[11] and the incidence of complete stent coverage was only 9.1% in SES and 29.6% in paclitaxel-eluting stent (PES; Taxus, Boston Scientific, Natick, MA, USA) at 9 months.[12] At serial follow-up with 6 months and ≥3 years, the percentage of uncovered struts decreased with SES (4.1% vs 0.9%, P = .002), but not with PES (3.2% vs 1.5%, P = .28).[16] However, another OCT study reported that there was no statistical difference in the percentage of uncovered struts between SES and PES at 5 years after implantation (1.5% vs 1.0%, P = .32).[14]

Several observational OCT studies suggest that second-generation DES are better than first-generation DES in terms of strut coverage. The Endeavor zotarolimus-eluting stent (Medtronic, Santa Rosa, CA, USA) showed near complete strut coverage (99.9%) at 3-month follow-up,[17] and the percentage of uncovered struts was lower with the Resolute zotarolimus-eluting stent (Medtronic) than with the Cypher stent at 9-month follow-up (4.4% vs 10.3%, P = .05).[18] At more than 12 months after implantation, the everolimus-eluting stent (Xience; Abbott Vascular, Abbott Park, IL, USA) displayed a lower percentage of uncovered struts compared with SES or PES (1.9% for Xience vs 11.6% for SES [P = .01] and vs 7.1% for PES [P<.001]).[19]

Randomized studies have confirmed these findings. At 6-month follow-up, the percentage of uncovered struts was lower with the biolimus-eluting stent (Nobori; Terumo Corp, Tokyo, Japan) than with SES (15.9% vs 25.1%, P = .003).[20] A serial OCT study demonstrated that the strut coverage of the Nobori stent was comparable with that of SES at 3 months, but at 1 year after stent implantation the Nobori stent showed better strut coverage than SES (percentage of uncovered struts 2.6% vs 6.2%, P = .028).[21] The strut coverage among second-generation DESs appeared comparable. The percentage of uncovered struts was not different between Resolute and Xience stents at 3-month follow-up (6.2% vs 4.7%, P = .62), and there also were no differences in coverage at 12 months.[22,23] These OCT findings are consistent with pathology studies, in that in human autopsies, everolimus-eluting stents demonstrate improved strut coverage with less inflammation,

less fibrin deposition, and less late and very late stent thrombosis in comparison with first-generation DES.[24]

The better strut coverage of second-generation DES seems to reduce the rate of late or very late stent thrombosis in comparison with first-generation DES. In the LEADERS trial, the biolimus-eluting stent (Biomatrix; Biosensors International, Singapore) improved the clinical safety compared with SES by reducing adverse cardiac events associated with very late stent thrombosis.[25,26] A prospective cohort study showed that everolimus-eluting stent implantation was directly related to the lower risk of stent thrombosis–associated events when compared with PES implantation (hazard ratio, 0.36; 95% confidence interval [CI], 0.23–0.57).[27] From the Swedish Coronary Angiography and Angioplasty Registry, second-generation DES including the Resolute zotarolimus-eluting stent and the everolimus-eluting stent were associated with a 43% lower risk of definite stent thrombosis and a 23% lower risk of death compared with first-generation DES.[28] Meta-analysis of randomized trials of primary percutaneous coronary intervention (PCI) also demonstrated lower incidence of stent thrombosis, myocardial infarction, and target vessel revascularization with second-generation DES when compared with BMS.[29]

The improvement of early strut coverage may reduce the duration of dual antiplatelet therapy. Although the current guideline recommends at least 12 months of aspirin and clopidogrel maintenance after DES deployment,[30] a randomized trial (RESET) showed the noninferiority of 3-month dual antiplatelet therapy after implantation of the Endeavor Sprint DES when compared with standard dual antiplatelet therapy (12 months) after implantation of other available DES.[31] In this study, the incidence of stent thrombosis was extremely low (0.2%–0.3%).[31] A meta-analysis including 4 randomized controlled trials demonstrated a nonsignificant higher rate of stent thrombosis in patients treated with a short course of dual antiplatelet therapy (0.35% vs 0.20%, P = .22),[32] whereas major bleeding was significantly higher in patients treated with prolonged dual antiplatelet therapy (0.29% vs 0.71%, P = .01).[32]

Recently, novel stents have been developed that consist of bioresorbable scaffolds. A pilot study demonstrated the feasibility of a polymeric bioresorbable DES in which the scaffolds disappear during follow-up.[33] This approach has several theoretic advantages by providing the short-term vessel scaffolding combined with drug delivery, restoring vasomotor function, and avoiding the permanent irritation of metallic stents. OCT has played a critical role in the evaluation of the natural history and vascular response to absorbable scaffolds, as these stent systems are not well visualized by intravascular ultrasonography. At 2 years after implantation of an everolimus-eluting bioresorbable scaffold, 34.5% of strut locations were no longer discernible by OCT, and the remaining struts were fully apposed.[34] Furthermore, late luminal enlargement resulting from plaque reduction was observed by OCT and intravascular ultrasonography.[34] In addition to polymeric scaffolds, a magnesium-based paclitaxel-eluting absorbable metal scaffold also showed promising performance up to 12 months.[35]

OTHER FACTORS AFFECTING STRUT COVERAGE

The clinical sequelae of stent malapposition have been hotly debated. An OCT study demonstrated that clinical events, including cardiovascular death, nonfatal myocardial infarction, and stent thrombosis, was not associated with OCT-detected late stent malapposition during a follow-up period of 28.6 ± 10.3 months.[36] Thus, from the data that are available it does not appear that OCT-detected stent malapposition is directly related to adverse cardiac events. However, stent malapposition may be a substrate for delayed neointimal healing. OCT has demonstrated that compared with well-apposed struts, malapposed struts are associated with a higher frequency of lack of coverage (**Fig. 2**).[37] Conversely, embedded struts after intervention demonstrate excellent coverage.[38] A study using computational fluid dynamics demonstrated positive relationships between malapposed distance, high peri-strut shear flow disturbances, and the frequency of uncovered struts,[39] thereby outlining a possible mechanism underlying the delayed healing observed with malapposition.

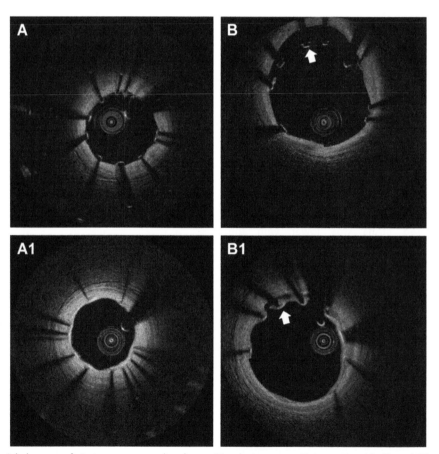

Fig. 2. Serial changes of strut coverage and malapposition between postintervention (*A, B*) and 12 months of follow-up (*A1, B1*). Well-apposed struts were fully covered on follow-up OCT (*A, A1*), whereas the coverage of struts with acute malapposition (*arrows*) was delayed. Malapposed struts with 630 μm of distance were partially integrated into the vessel wall (*B, B1*).

OCT imaging demonstrates that early or acute stent malapposition (ie, immediately after PCI) is a common phenomenon, occurring in as many as 62% of stented lesions. However, about two-thirds of this malapposition is completely resolved by approximately 1 year after implantation.[36,40,41] Several predictors of persistent malapposition have been identified by OCT studies (Box 1). An important predictor of the resolution of malapposed struts is the magnitude of malapposition (measured by the volume of malapposition or malapposed strut-to-vessel distance).[36,40–42] The optimal cutoff point for strut-to-vessel distance to predict resolution was 280 µm or less for SES (sensitivity 95.0%, specificity 100%, area under the curve [AUC] = 0.991), 260 µm or less for PES (sensitivity 87.8%, specificity 80.0%, AUC = 0.865), and 380 µm or less for everolimus-eluting stents (sensitivity 93.5%, specificity 69.8%, AUC = 0.878).[41,42] Another OCT-derived predictor for persistent stent malapposition is the location of stent malapposition within the stent edges.[36] Clinical factors may also affect the strut coverage after DES implantation. Several OCT studies have demonstrated an association between strut coverage and clinical presentation, the character of underlying plaque, and the statin usage. Uncovered struts were more frequently observed among patients with acute coronary syndrome than in those with stable coronary artery disease (1.7% vs 0.7%, adjusted $P = .041$).[43] Acute stent malapposition remained persistent more frequently over lipid/calcified than over fibrous plaques, even when the strut-to-vessel distance was small.[42] Malapposed and uncovered struts were less frequently detected in patients receiving rosuvastatin than in those with pravastatin (malapposed, 0.06% vs 0.60%, $P<.001$; uncovered, 6.49% vs 11.29%, $P<.001$).[44]

CONTOUR PLOT ANALYSIS

Contour plot analysis is a comprehensive approach to analyze the status of stent struts over time.[45] A contour plot is a graphic representation of the associations among 3 numeric variables in 2 dimensions. In the contour plot of coronary stent struts, x and y axes represent circumferential arc length and stent length, respectively. A third variable, z, represents neointimal thickness or strut-to-vessel distance as contour level. The contour plot analysis enables the simultaneous demonstration of both strut coverage and apposition, and highlights the status or changes of stent struts (Fig. 3). An OCT study showed that the Nobori stent had a lower incidence of diffuse distribution pattern of uncovered struts when compared with SES.[20] In addition, serial tracking using contour plots demonstrated that embedded and apposed struts after intervention had a higher rate of strut coverage at 6-month follow-up than was observed in malapposed struts.[38]

OPTICAL COHERENCE TOMOGRAPHY– GUIDED OPTIMIZATION OF STENT IMPLANTATION

OCT guidance for PCI may substantially improve strut coverage by reducing the stent malapposition. A randomized study compared strut coverage and apposition between angiographic- and OCT-guided PCI using the Resolute zotarolimus-eluting stent.[46] At 6-month follow-up, the percentage of uncovered struts was significantly lower with OCT guidance when compared with angiographic guidance (1.60% vs 4.51%, $P = .0004$). The percentage of malapposed struts was also lower in the OCT-guided group (0.19% vs 0.98%, $P = .027$).[46] In another study using multivariable and propensity-score adjusted analysis, angiographic plus OCT-guided PCI was associated with a lower risk of cardiac death or myocardial infarction (odds ratio, 0.49; 95% CI, 0.25–0.96) compared with angiographically guided PCI alone.[47]

NEOATHEROSCLEROSIS

Normal neointima is mainly composed of smooth muscle cells and extracellular matrix, and is homogeneously characterized by strong optical intensity and mild attenuation rate on OCT.[48] However, recent pathologic, angioscopic, and OCT studies have demonstrated the presence of atherosclerosis within the neointima of both BMS and DES, a phenomenon termed neoatherosclerosis. Fig. 4 illustrates an

---

Box 1
Predictors of persistent strut malapposition in optical coherence studies of drug-eluting stents

Strut-to-vessel distance

Total volume of malapposition

Location of malapposition along stent length

Acute coronary syndrome presentation

Intensive statin use

Lipid/calcified plaque

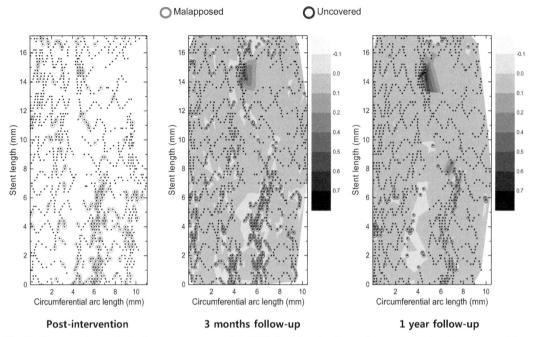

Fig. 3. Contour plot analysis of coronary stents using OCT. Serial evaluations using contour plot demonstrated that malapposed struts (*red circles*) spontaneously resolved after drug-stent implantation. However, uncovered struts (*blue circles*) were frequently observed in the portion of malapposed struts during serial follow-up.

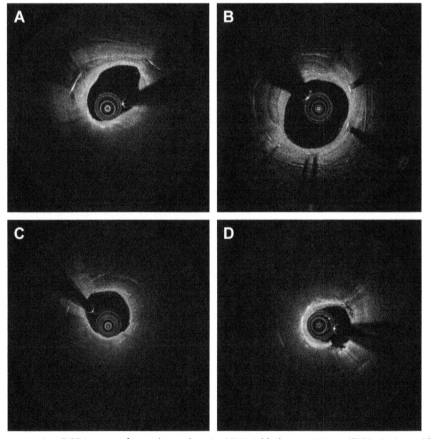

Fig. 4. Representative OCT images of neoatherosclerosis. (*A*) Lipid-laden neointima. (*B*) Neointima with calcification. (*C*) Thin-cap fibroatheroma-like neointima. (*D*) Neointimal rupture.

example of neoatherosclerosis identified by OCT. Neoatherosclerosis has been observed in both BMS and DES, but develops earlier within DES than in BMS: in a human autopsy study, the median stent duration with neoatherosclerosis was 420 days after DES compared with 2160 days after BMS.[49] Unstable features such as thin-cap fibroatheroma or plaque rupture are associated with neoatherosclerosis.[49]

Several in vivo OCT studies have investigated the incidence, predictors, and clinical outcomes of neoatherosclerosis. In the first 48 months after stent implantation, the incidence of lipid-laden neointima is higher in DES than in BMS.[50] However, after 48 months the incidence was similar between stent types.[50] Another OCT study found that neoatherosclerotic neointima was commonly observed in DES-treated lesions with greater than 50% of neointimal cross-sectional area stenosis and more than 30 months of stent duration.[51] Serial OCT studies have documented the development of neoatherosclerosis: from 9 months to 2 years post-DES, the frequency of lipid-laden neointima increased from 14.5% to 27.6% ($P =$ .009), as did the frequency of thin-cap fibroatheroma (from 3.9% to 13.2%, $P = $ .07).[52] In matched serial follow-up evaluations, neoatherosclerotic change of neointimal tissue was associated with a significant increase of neointimal burden.[53]

Several risk factors for neoatherosclerosis have been identified. Younger age, longer implant durations, use of first-generation DES, and underlying unstable plaques were independent determinants for neoatherosclerosis according to a human pathology study.[49] One OCT study suggested that more than 48 months of stent duration, all subtypes of DES (compared with BMS), current smoking, chronic kidney disease, and angiotensin-converting enzyme inhibitors/angiotensin receptor blockade use were predictors for neoatherosclerosis.[54] Another OCT study reported that stent duration, hypertension, and the use of first-generation DES (compared with BMS) were risk factors.[51] Lesion-specific factors might be also associated with neoatherosclerotic changes: neoatherosclerosis occurred more frequently at the proximal or distal segment of the implanted stent, and was related to adjacent de novo lipid-laden plaque.[55] This latter finding suggests that there may be an important interaction between de novo plaques and the development of adjacent neoatherosclerosis within the stent.

Neoatherosclerosis contributes to progressive neointimal hyperplasia and deteriorates the clinical presentation, irrespective of BMS or DES. In BMS restenotic lesions, the proportions of cross sections with heterogeneous intima (including neoatherosclerosis) in the entire stent were significantly higher in the late-ISR group than in the early-ISR group (60.5% ± 28.5% vs 5.8% ± 11.5%, $P<.0001$)[56]; a similar pattern was observed in DES restenosis.[57] Compared with patients presenting with stable angina, those with unstable angina showed a higher frequency of unstable OCT findings such as thin-cap fibroatheroma-containing neointima, neointimal rupture, and thrombus.[58] In addition, the incidence of target-lesion revascularization or stent thrombosis was common in patients with neoatherosclerotic in-stent restenosis.[51] Therefore, the presence of neoatherosclerosis could explain the steady increase of stent thrombosis over time, and may be a key mechanism underlying late stent failure and late stent thrombosis.[59] In addition, neoatherosclerosis may influence procedural outcomes for the treatment of in-stent restenosis, as in-stent thin-cap fibroatheroma was also more prevalent in patients with periprocedural myocardial infarction than in those without.[60]

CHARACTERISTICS OF NEOINTIMA WITHOUT FEATURES OF NEOATHEROSCLEROSIS DETECTED BY OPTICAL COHERENCE TOMOGRAPHY

Besides neoatherosclerosis, various types of neointimal tissues can be differentiated by OCT. An OCT study categorized restenotic neointimal tissue into 3 types: (1) homogeneous, uniform optical properties without focal variations in backscattering pattern; (2) heterogeneous, focally changing optical properties with various backscattering patterns; and (3) layered, concentric optical properties with adluminal high and abluminal low scattering layers (Fig. 5).[61] Although there has been a lack of histologic data to validate this classification, the low optical intensity area of restenosis was associated with myxomatous tissue or fibrin thrombus.[62] A recent study showed that adverse cardiac events occurred more frequently in patients with heterogeneous neointima when compared with nonheterogeneous neointima during the average 31 months of follow-up.[63] In another report, the mechanism of postintervention lumen enlargement by drug-eluting balloon angioplasty for DES in-stent restenotic lesions varied with preintervention OCT-based neointimal characteristics, and in-stent restenotic lesions with homogeneous neointima were associated with greater subsequent regrowth of neointima at follow-up OCT.[64]

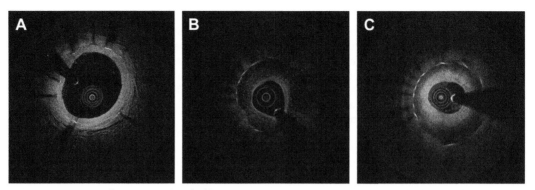

Fig. 5. Various types of neointima identified by OCT. (*A*) Homogeneous neointima. (*B*) Heterogeneous neointima. (*C*) Layered neointima.

LIMITATIONS OF OPTICAL COHERENCE TOMOGRAPHY

Several limitations should be considered when interpreting OCT studies. OCT-defined coverage of stent struts does not always mean true neointima. Although a pathologic study validated that OCT-derived identification of individual uncovered struts showed sensitivity of 77.9% and specificity of 96.4%,[48] the current OCT system cannot discriminate true neointima from fibrin deposits, especially in the early phase after stent implantation. Because lipid, peri-strut inflammation, fibrin deposit, and abundant extracellular matrix within neointima similarly appear dark on OCT,[48] the characterization of neointimal tissue by OCT may be misleading in some cases. Because OCT has low penetration depth, the external elastic membrane of lesions of interest occasionally cannot be evaluated.

SUMMARY

OCT evaluation has revealed novel findings regarding the natural history of strut coverage and neointimal development after DES implantation. Strut coverage has improved with the second generation of DES, and subsequently the incidence of stent thrombosis has decreased. The improved coverage of new DES might reduce the duration of dual antiplatelet therapy, although this remains to be robustly studied. Several risk factors for persistent malapposition, which is associated with delayed healing, can be identified with OCT. As significant volume or distance of stent malapposition is associated with persistent lack of coverage, a stent optimization strategy using OCT guidance might have clinical benefit. During the late phase of post–stent implantation, neoatherosclerosis contributes to progressive neointimal growth and increases the vulnerability of neointimal tissue to contribute to acute ischemic or thrombotic events. Besides neoatherosclerosis, the various types of neointimal tissue identified on OCT are also under investigation.

REFERENCES

1. Lee SY, Hong MK. Stent evaluation with optical coherence tomography. Yonsei Med J 2013;54: 1075–83.
2. Suzuki Y, Ikeno F, Koizumi T, et al. In vivo comparison between optical coherence tomography and intravascular ultrasound for detecting small degrees of in-stent neointima after stent implantation. JACC Cardiovasc Interv 2008;1:168–73.
3. Kwon SW, Kim BK, Kim TH, et al. Qualitative assessment of neointimal tissue after drug-eluting stent implantation: comparison between follow-up optical coherence tomography and intravascular ultrasound. Am Heart J 2011;161:367–72.
4. Takarada S, Imanishi T, Liu Y, et al. Advantage of next-generation frequency-domain optical coherence tomography compared with conventional time-domain system in the assessment of coronary lesion. Catheter Cardiovasc Interv 2010;75:202–6.
5. Forrester JS, Fishbein M, Helfant R, et al. A paradigm for restenosis based on cell biology: clues for the development of new preventive therapies. J Am Coll Cardiol 1991;17:758–69.
6. Joner M, Finn AV, Farb A, et al. Pathology of drug-eluting stents in humans: delayed healing and late thrombotic risk. J Am Coll Cardiol 2006;48:193–202.
7. Finn AV, Kolodgie FD, Harnek J, et al. Differential response of delayed healing and persistent inflammation at sites of overlapping sirolimus- or paclitaxel-eluting stents. Circulation 2005;112:270–8.
8. Finn AV, Joner M, Nakazawa G, et al. Pathological correlates of late drug-eluting stent thrombosis: strut coverage as a marker of endothelialization. Circulation 2007;115:2435–41.

9. Guagliumi G, Sirbu V, Musumeci G, et al. Examination of the in vivo mechanisms of late drug-eluting stent thrombosis: findings from optical coherence tomography and intravascular ultrasound imaging. JACC Cardiovasc Interv 2012;5:12–20.

10. Won H, Shin DH, Kim BK, et al. Optical coherence tomography derived cut-off value of uncovered stent struts to predict adverse clinical outcomes after drug-eluting stent implantation. Int J Cardiovasc Imaging 2013;29:1–9.

11. Matsumoto D, Shite J, Shinke T, et al. Neointimal coverage of sirolimus-eluting stents at 6-month follow-up: evaluated by optical coherence tomography. Eur Heart J 2007;28:961–7.

12. Kim J, Kim TH, Fan C, et al. Comparison of neointimal coverage of sirolimus-eluting stents and paclitaxel-eluting stents using optical coherence tomography at 9 months after implantation. Circ J 2010;74:320–6.

13. Kim T, Kim J, Kim B, et al. Long-term (≥2 years) follow-up optical coherence tomographic study after sirolimus- and paclitaxel-eluting stent implantation: comparison to 9-month follow-up results. Int J Cardiovasc Imaging 2011;27:875–81.

14. Räber L, Baumgartner S, Garcia-Garcia HM, et al. Long-term vascular healing in response to sirolimus- and paclitaxel-eluting stents: an optical coherence tomography study. JACC Cardiovasc Interv 2012;5:946–57.

15. Nakamura D, Lee Y, Yoshimura T, et al. Different serial changes in the neointimal condition of sirolimus-eluting stents and paclitaxel-eluting stents: an optical coherence tomographic study. EuroIntervention 2014;10(8):924–33.

16. Nakagawa M, Otake H, Shinke T, et al. Analysis by optical coherence tomography of long-term arterial healing after implantation of different types of stents. Can J Cardiol 2014;30(8):904–11.

17. Kim J, Jang I, Fan C, et al. Evaluation in 3 months duration of neointimal coverage after zotarolimus-eluting stent implantation by optical coherence tomography: the ENDEAVOR OCT trial. JACC Cardiovasc Interv 2009;2:1240–7.

18. Kim J, Shin D, Kim B, et al. Optical coherence tomographic comparison of neointimal coverage between sirolimus- and resolute zotarolimus-eluting stents at 9 months after stent implantation. Int J Cardiovasc Imaging 2012;28:1281–7.

19. Toledano Delgado FJ, Alvarez-Ossorio MP, de Lezo Cruz-Conde JS, et al. Optical coherence tomography evaluation of late strut coverage patterns between first-generation drug-eluting stents and everolimus-eluting stent. Catheter Cardiovasc Interv 2014;84(5):720–6.

20. Kim BK, Ha J, Mintz GS, et al. Randomised comparison of strut coverage between Nobori biolimus-eluting and sirolimus-eluting stents: an optical coherence tomography analysis. EuroIntervention 2014;9:1389–97.

21. Kim BK, Hong MK, Shin DH, et al. Optical coherence tomography analysis of strut coverage in biolimus- and sirolimus-eluting stents: 3-month and 12-month serial follow-up. Int J Cardiol 2013; 168:4617–23.

22. Kim S, Kim J, Shin D, et al. Comparison of early strut coverage between zotarolimus- and everolimus-eluting stents using optical coherence tomography. Am J Cardiol 2013;111:1–5.

23. Gutiérrez-Chico JL, van Geuns RJ, Regar E, et al. Tissue coverage of a hydrophilic polymer-coated zotarolimus-eluting stent vs a fluoropolymer-coated everolimus-eluting stent at 13-month follow-up: an optical coherence tomography substudy from the RESOLUTE All Comers trial. Eur Heart J 2011;32:2454–63.

24. Otsuka F, Vorpahl M, Nakano M, et al. Pathology of second-generation everolimus-eluting stents versus first-generation sirolimus- and paclitaxel-eluting stents in humans. Circulation 2014;129: 211–23.

25. Windecker S, Serruys PW, Wandel S, et al. Biolimus-eluting stent with biodegradable polymer versus sirolimus-eluting stent with durable polymer for coronary revascularisation (LEADERS): a randomised non-inferiority trial. Lancet 2008;372: 1163–73.

26. Stefanini G, Kalesan B, Serruys PW, et al. Long-term clinical outcomes of biodegradable polymer biolimus-eluting stents versus durable polymer sirolimus-eluting stents in patients with coronary artery disease (LEADERS): 4 year follow-up of a randomised non-inferiority trial. Lancet 2011;378: 1940–8.

27. Räber L, Magro M, Stefanini G, et al. Very late coronary stent thrombosis of a newer-generation everolimus-eluting stent compared with early-generation drug-eluting stents: a prospective cohort study. Circulation 2012;125:1110–21.

28. Sarno G, Lagerqvist B, Fröbert O, et al. Lower risk of stent thrombosis and restenosis with unrestricted use of 'new-generation' drug-eluting stents: a report from the nationwide Swedish Coronary Angiography and Angioplasty Registry (SCAAR). Eur Heart J 2012;33:606–13.

29. Philip F, Agarwal S, Bunte MC, et al. Stent thrombosis with second-generation drug-eluting stents compared with bare-metal stents: network meta-analysis of primary percutaneous coronary intervention trials in ST-segment-elevation myocardial infarction. Circ Cardiovasc Interv 2014;7:49–61.

30. Smith SC Jr, Benjamin EJ, Bonow RO, et al. AHA/ACCF secondary prevention and risk reduction therapy for patients with coronary and other atherosclerotic vascular disease: 2011 update: a

guideline from the American Heart Association and American College of Cardiology Foundation endorsed by the World Heart Federation and the Preventive Cardiovascular Nurses Association. J Am Coll Cardiol 2011;58:2432–46.

31. Kim BK, Hong MK, Shin DH, et al. A new strategy for discontinuation of dual antiplatelet therapy: the RESET Trial (REal Safety and Efficacy of 3-month dual antiplatelet Therapy following Endeavor zotarolimus-eluting stent implantation). J Am Coll Cardiol 2012;60:1340–8.

32. El-Hayek G, Messerli F, Bangalore S, et al. Meta-analysis of randomized clinical trials comparing short-term versus long-term dual antiplatelet therapy following drug-eluting stents. Am J Cardiol 2014;114:236–42.

33. Ormiston JA, Serruys PW, Regar E, et al. A bioabsorbable everolimus-eluting coronary stent system for patients with single de-novo coronary artery lesions (ABSORB): a prospective open-label trial. Lancet 2008;371:899–907.

34. Serruys PW, Ormiston JA, Onuma Y, et al. A bioabsorbable everolimus-eluting coronary stent system (ABSORB): 2-year outcomes and results from multiple imaging methods. Lancet 2009;373: 897–910.

35. Haude M, Erbel R, Erne P, et al. Safety and performance of the drug-eluting absorbable metal scaffold (DREAMS) in patients with de-novo coronary lesions: 12 month results of the prospective, multicentre, first-in-man BIOSOLVE-I trial. Lancet 2013; 381:836–44.

36. Im E, Kim BK, Ko YG, et al. Incidences, predictors, and clinical outcomes of acute and late stent malapposition detected by optical coherence tomography after drug-eluting stent implantation. Circ Cardiovasc Interv 2014;7:88–96.

37. GutiÃrrez-Chico JL, Regar E, Nesch E, et al. Delayed coverage in malapposed and side-branch struts with respect to well-apposed struts in drug-eluting stents: in vivo assessment with optical coherence tomography. Circulation 2011;124: 612–23.

38. Kim JS, Ha J, Kim BK, et al. The relationship between post-stent strut apposition and follow-up strut coverage assessed by a contour plot optical coherence tomography analysis. JACC Cardiovasc Interv 2014;7:641–51.

39. Foin N, GutiÃrrez-Chico JL, Nakatani S, et al. Incomplete stent apposition causes high shear flow disturbances and delay in neointimal coverage as a function of strut to wall detachment distance: implications for the management of incomplete stent apposition. Circ Cardiovasc Interv 2014;7: 180–9.

40. GutiÃrrez-Chico JL, Wykrzykowska J, Nüesch E, et al. Vascular tissue reaction to acute malapposition in human coronary arteries: sequential assessment with optical coherence tomography. Circ Cardiovasc Interv 2012;5:20–9.

41. Kawamori H, Shite J, Shinke T, et al. Natural consequence of post-intervention stent malapposition, thrombus, tissue prolapse, and dissection assessed by optical coherence tomography at mid-term follow-up. Eur Heart J Cardiovasc Imaging 2013; 14:865–75.

42. Inoue T, Shinke T, Otake H, et al. Impact of strut-vessel distance and underlying plaque type on the resolution of acute strut malapposition: serial optimal coherence tomography analysis after everolimus-eluting stent implantation. Int J Cardiovasc Imaging 2014;30:857–65.

43. Räber L, Zanchin T, Baumgartner S, et al. Differential healing response attributed to culprit lesions of patients with acute coronary syndromes and stable coronary artery after implantation of drug-eluting stents: an optical coherence tomography study. Int J Cardiol 2014;173:259–67.

44. Yamamoto H, Ikuta S, Kobuke K, et al. Difference in statin effects on neointimal coverage after implantation of drug-eluting stents. Coron Artery Dis 2014;25:290–5.

45. Ha J, Kim BK, Kim JS, et al. A new method for assessing neointimal coverage after drug-eluting stent implantation using three-dimensional optical coherence tomography. J Am Coll Cardiol Img 2012;5: 852–3. Available at: http://jaccjacc.cardiosource. com/DataSupp/JCMG_Author_Instructions_060914. pdf.

46. Kim JS, Shin DH, Kim BK, et al. Randomized comparison of stent strut coverage following angiography- or optical coherence tomography-guided percutaneous coronary intervention. Rev Esp Cardiol (Engl Ed) 2015;68(3):190–7.

47. Prati F, Di Vito L, Biondi-Zoccai G, et al. Angiography alone versus angiography plus optical coherence tomography to guide decision-making during percutaneous coronary intervention: the Centro per la Lotta contro l'Infarto-Optimisation of Percutaneous Coronary Intervention (CLI-OPCI) study. EuroIntervention 2012;8:823–9.

48. Nakano M, Vorpahl M, Otsuka F, et al. Ex vivo assessment of vascular response to coronary stents by optical frequency domain imaging. JACC Cardiovasc Imaging 2012;5:71–82.

49. Nakazawa G, Otsuka F, Nakano M, et al. The pathology of neoatherosclerosis in human coronary implants bare-metal and drug-eluting stents. J Am Coll Cardiol 2011;57:1314–22.

50. Yonetsu T, Kim JS, Kato K, et al. Comparison of incidence and time course of neoatherosclerosis between bare metal stents and drug-eluting stents using optical coherence tomography. Am J Cardiol 2012;110:933–9.

51. Lee SY, Shin DH, Mintz GS, et al. Optical coherence tomography-based evaluation of in-stent neoatherosclerosis in lesions with more than 50% neointimal cross-sectional area stenosis. EuroIntervention 2013;9:945–51.

52. Kim JS, Hong MK, Shin DH, et al. Quantitative and qualitative changes in DES-related neointimal tissue based on serial OCT. JACC Cardiovasc Imaging 2012;5:1147–55.

53. Lee SY, Hong MK, Mintz GS, et al. Temporal course of neointimal hyperplasia following drug-eluting stent implantation: a serial follow-up optical coherence tomography analysis. Int J Cardiovasc Imaging 2014;30:1003–11.

54. Yonetsu T, Kato K, Kim SJ, et al. Predictors for neoatherosclerosis: a retrospective observational study from the optical coherence tomography registry. Circ Cardiovasc Imaging 2012;5:660–6.

55. Tian J, Ren X, Uemura S, et al. Spatial heterogeneity of neoatherosclerosis and its relationship with neovascularization and adjacent plaque characteristics: optical coherence tomography study. Am Heart J 2014;167:884–92.

56. Habara M, Terashima M, Nasu K, et al. Difference of tissue characteristics between early and very late restenosis lesions after bare-metal stent implantation: an optical coherence tomography study. Circ Cardiovasc Interv 2011;4:232–8.

57. Habara M, Terashima M, Nasu K, et al. Morphological differences of tissue characteristics between early, late, and very late restenosis lesions after first generation drug-eluting stent implantation: an optical coherence tomography study. Eur Heart J Cardiovasc Imaging 2012;14:276–84.

58. Kang SJ, Mintz GS, Akasaka T, et al. Optical coherence tomographic analysis of in-stent neoatherosclerosis after drug-eluting stent implantation. Circulation 2011;123:2954–63.

59. Park S, Kang S, Virmani R, et al. In-stent neoatherosclerosis: a final common pathway of late stent failure. J Am Coll Cardiol 2012;59:2051–7.

60. Ali ZA, Roleder T, Narula J, et al. Increased thin-cap neoatheroma and periprocedural myocardial infarction in drug-eluting stent restenosis: multimodality intravascular imaging of drug-eluting and bare-metal stents. Circ Cardiovasc Interv 2013;6:507–17.

61. Gonzalo N, Serruys PW, Okamura T, et al. Optical coherence tomography patterns of stent restenosis. Am Heart J 2009;158:284–93.

62. Kim JS, Afari ME, Ha J, et al. Neointimal patterns obtained by optical coherence tomography correlate with specific histological components and neointimal proliferation in a swine model of restenosis. Eur Heart J Cardiovasc Imaging 2014;15:292–8.

63. Kim JS, Lee JH, Shin DH, et al. Long-term outcomes of neointimal hyperplasia without features of neoatherosclerosis after drug-eluting stent implantation. JACC Cardiovasc Imaging 2014;7(8): 788–95.

64. Lee SY, Hong MK, Shin DH, et al. Mechanisms of postintervention and nine-month luminal enlargement after treatment of drug-eluting in-stent restenosis with a drug-eluting balloon. Am J Cardiol 2014;113:1468–73.

Short- and Long-term Evaluation of Bioresorbable Scaffolds by Optical Coherence Tomography

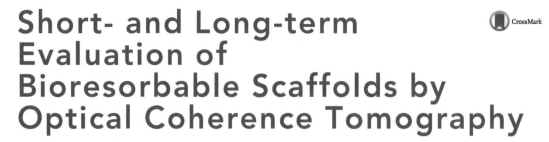 CrossMark

Carlos M. Campos, MD[a,b], Pannipa Suwannasom, MD[a],
Shimpei Nakatani, MD[a], Yoshinobu Onuma, MD, PhD[a],
Patrick W. Serruys, MD, PhD[a,c],
Hector M. Garcia-Garcia, MD, PhD[a,d,*]

KEYWORDS

- Bioresorbable scaffolds • Optical coherence tomography • Drug-eluting stents

---

KEY POINTS

- The analysis of bioresorbable scaffolds (BRSs) by optical coherence tomography (OCT) requires a dedicated methodology, as the polymeric scaffold has a distinct appearance and undergoes dynamic structural changes with time, unlike metallic stents.
- The high resolution of OCT allows for the detailed assessment of scaffold implantation, rupture, discontinuity, and strut integration.
- OCT does not provide reliable information on the extent of scaffold degradation, as it cannot differentiate between polylactide polymer and the provisional matrix of proteoglycan formed by connective tissue.
- Three-dimensional OCT reconstruction can aid in the evaluation of BRS in special scenarios such as overlapping scaffold segments and bifurcations.

INTRODUCTION

BRSs represent a novel approach in the treatment of coronary artery disease. They support the vessel transiently to maintain patency after intervention, deliver antiproliferative drug to the vessel wall, and then gradually degrade.[1,2] BRS technology has matured, and there are numerous devices that are commercially available outside the United States or are undergoing preclinical or clinical evaluation (Fig. 1). BRS has required new imaging modalities, methodologies, and strategies, because

scaffold design, degradation rate, loss of mechanical properties (Table 1), coating, and drug deliverability may affect BRS safety and efficacy.[3,4] OCT has played a central role in understanding the short and long term BRS performance, OCT provides more detailed and precise morphologic information about BRS than does intravascular ultrasonography (IVUS) because of its higher resolution.[5,6] This review summarizes the methodology and clinical application of OCT in the assessment of BRS, in particular for the commercially available Absorb Bioresorbable

---

The authors have nothing to disclose.

[a] Department of Interventional Cardiology, Thoraxcenter, Erasmus University Medical Centre, Dr. Molewaterplein 40, Rotterdam 3015 GD, The Netherlands; [b] Department of Interventional Cardiology Heart Institute (InCor), University of São Paulo Medical School, Avenida Doutor Enéas de Carvalho Aguiar, 44 - Terceiro Andar, Sao Paulo 05403-900, Brazil; [c] International Centre for Circulatory Health, National Heart and Lung Institute, Imperial College London, South Kensington Campus, London SW7 2AZ, UK; [d] Medical Affairs, Cardialysis, Westblaak 98, Entrance B, Rotterdam 3012 KM, The Netherlands
* Corresponding author. Westblaak 98, Entrance B, Rotterdam 3012 KM, The Netherlands.
E-mail address: h.garciagarcia@erasmusmc.nl

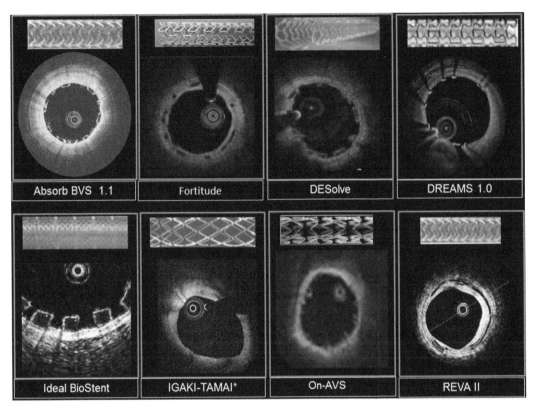

Fig. 1. Optical coherence tomography images of different bioresorbable vascular scaffolds. Absorb BVS 1.1 (Abbott Vascular, Santa Clara, CA, USA); Fortitude (Amaranth Medical, Mountain View, CA, USA); DESolve BRS (Elixir, Sunnyvale, CA, USA); DREAMS 1.0 absorbable metallic scaffold (Biotronik, Berlin, Germany); Ideal II BioStent (Xenogenics, Philadelphia, PA, USA); Igaki-Tamai scaffold (Kyoto Medical Planning Co, Kyoto, Japan); On-AVS (Orbus Neich, Wanchai, Hong Kong); REVA (REVA Medical Inc, San Diego, CA, USA). An OCT image for Igaki-Tamai was not available at baseline.

Table 1
Mechanical properties and degradation rate of different material candidates for bioresorbable coronary scaffolds

Material	Tensile Strength (MPa)	Elongation (%)	Degradation Time
Poly(L-lactide)	60–70	2–6	24 mo[a]
Poly(DL-lactide)	45–55	2–6	12–16 mo[a]
Poly(glycolide)	90–110	1–2	6–12 mo[a]
50/50 DL-lactide/glycolide	40–50	1–4	1–2 mo[a]
82/18 L-lactide/glycolide	60–70	2–6	12–18 mo[a]
70/30 L-lactide/ε-aprolactone	18–22	>100	12–24 mo[a]
Pure Fe	200	40	0.19 mm/y
Fe-35 Mn alloy	430	30	0.44 mm/y
WE43 alloy	280	2	1.35 mm/y

[a] Degradation time depends on geometry.
Data from Moravej M, Mantovani D. Biodegradable metals for cardiovascular stent application: interests and new opportunities. Int J Mol Sci 2011;12:4250–70; and van Alst M, Eenink MJ, Kruft MA, et al. ABC's of bioabsorption: application of lactide based polymers in fully resorbable cardiovascular stents. EuroIntervention 2009;5(Suppl F):F23–7.

Vascular Scaffold (BVS) (Abbot Vascular, Santa Clara, CA, USA), as this device had the most extensive short- and long-term follow-up data.

RATIONALE FOR THE NEED FOR A DEDICATED ANALYSIS METHODOLOGY FOR THE OPTICAL COHERENCE TOMOGRAPHIC ASSESSMENT OF BIORESORBABLE SCAFFOLDS

The OCT appearance of polymeric scaffolds differs significantly from that of metallic scaffolds and stents (Fig. 2A). The appearance of magnesium scaffolds immediately after implantation is similar to that of a permanent metallic stent, that is, a bright strut with well-delimited borders with a shadow behind (see Fig. 2A). In contradistinction, polymeric struts are optically translucent and appear as a black central core framed by light-scattering borders that do not shadow the vessel wall, and therefore the complete thickness of the scaffold strut can be visualized (see Fig. 2B). The main quantitative measurements for scaffold evaluation by OCT include strut core area, strut area, lumen area, scaffold area, incomplete strut apposition (ISA) area, and neointimal area. Because polymeric scaffolds scatter light differently and have different OCT characteristics than metallic stents/scaffolds (see Fig. 2B, C), these measurements must be acquired using different image analysis rules.

OPTICAL COHERENCE TOMOGRAPHIC EVALUATION OF BIORESORBABLE SCAFFOLDS AT TIME OF IMPLANTATION

Several OCT parameters can be collected at the time of short-term implantation of the BRS; these are summarized in Table 2. Key quantifications include the lumen and scaffold areas, the magnitude of ISA, lumen prolapse, and flow area. The high resolution provided by OCT also allows the operator to visualize the quality of scaffold implantation and the potential complications related to it. Important analyses include assessments of short-term strut fracture, edge dissection, eccentricity, and symmetry.

Contours
At baseline, the lumen and scaffold contours are obtained with a semiautomated detection algorithm available in numerous off-line software packages. These contours can be corrected manually if necessary.

Lumen and Scaffold Areas
Because the polymeric struts are translucent, the vessel lumen border can be visualized and the

vessel lumen area delineated along the external (abluminal) side of the struts. The scaffold area is measured by joining the internal middle points of the abluminal side of the black cores of the apposed struts or the abluminal edge of the frame borders of malapposed struts. In the absence of ISA and plaque prolapse, the scaffold area is identical to the lumen area (see Fig. 2C).

Incomplete Strut Apposition
ISA is defined by a clear separation between the abluminal side of the strut and the vessel wall. ISA area is delineated by the abluminal side of the frame border of the malapposed struts and the endoluminal contour of the lumen.

Lumen Prolapse
Several different parameters can be collected in the case of lumen or plaque prolapse protruding between the struts into the lumen. The prolapse area can be estimated by the planimetered difference between the prolapsed contour (ie, lumen contour) and the scaffold area. An intraluminal defect that is separated from the vessel wall (eg, thrombus) can also be quantified as an area.

Flow Area
Flow area takes into account ISA, plaque prolapse, and intraluminal defects. It is defined as the difference between the sum of the scaffold and ISA areas and the sum of the areas of intraluminal struts, prolapse, and intraluminal defect (ie, flow area = [scaffold area + ISA area] − [intraluminal strut areas + prolapse area + intraluminal defect area]).

Short-term Strut Fracture
The diagnosis of short-term strut fracture due to balloon overdilation can be established if 2 struts overhang each other within the same angular sector of the lumen perimeter (Fig. 3). This complication may be observed with or without concomitant strut malapposition. However, if isolated struts are located more or less at the center of the vessel without an obvious connection with other surrounding struts, strut fracture may also be present. It is helpful to perform 3-dimensional reconstruction of the OCT dataset to confirm the diagnosis.

Edge Dissection
Edge dissection is defined by OCT as the disruption of the endoluminal vessel surface at the proximal and distal edges of the BRS (Fig. 4).[7] In the ABSORB Cohort B trial, 24% of patients had proximal and 42% had distal edge dissection flaps postprocedure.[8] On follow-up, proximal and distal edge dissection flaps seem to

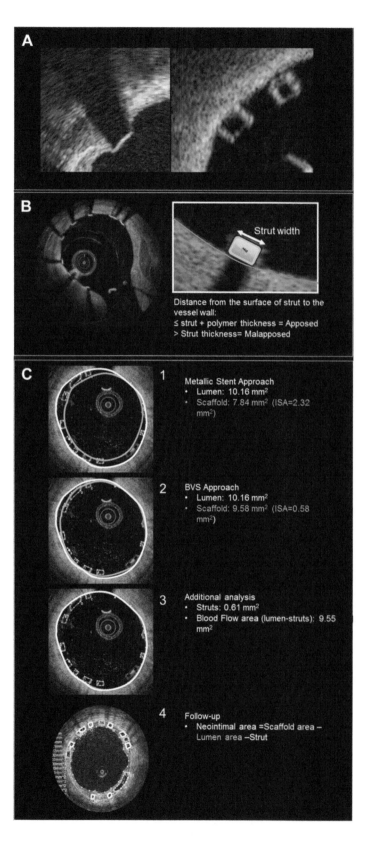

Fig. 2. (A) Representative optical coherence tomographic image of the drug-eluting absorbable metal scaffold DREAMS (Biotronik, Bülach, Switzerland) immediately after implantation looks like a permanent metallic stent (left). Absorb BVS has optically translucent struts and appears as a black central core framed by light-scattering borders that do not shadow the vessel wall and allow complete imaging of the strut thickness (right). (B) Methodology for the assessment of incomplete scaffold apposition (ISA) with the drug-eluting absorbable metal scaffold DREAMS. (C) Newly implanted bioresorbable scaffold. Differences in the methodology of OCT assessment between metallic stents and BVS are illustrated. Panel 1. Metallic stent approach. Note that with metallic scaffold/stent analysis, device area is calculated by planimetry of the endoluminal border of the struts. Lumen area, 10.16 mm²; stent area, 7.84 mm², ISA, 2.32 mm². Panel 2. BVS approach. Lumen area, 10.16 mm²; stent area, 9.58 mm²; ISA, 0.58 mm². Panel 3. Additional BVS analyses. Strut area, 0.61 mm²; blood flow area (lumen area − strut area), 9.55 mm². Panel 4. Follow-up OCT imaging of BVS. Strut area is defined only by its black core, because the light-scattering frame is no longer distinguishable from the surrounding tissue. Neointimal area is defined by (scaffold area − lumen area − strut area). ([C] Adapted from Garcia-Garcia HM, Serruys PW, Campos CM, et al. Assessing bioresorbable coronary devices: methods and parameters. JACC Cardiovasc Imaging 2014;7:1130–48.)

Table 2
Definitions and formulas for the quantification of OCT parameters for the assessment of BRSs

Parameter	Formula	Definition and Notes
Eccentricity index	Minimum scaffold diameter/maximum scaffold diameter in a frame	The average of all eccentricity indices of each frame within scaffolded segment is calculated
Symmetry index	(Minimum scaffold diameter − maximum scaffold diameter)/ maximum scaffold diameter within a scaffolded segment	The maximum and the minimum stent/scaffold diameters in this calculation were possibly located in 2 different frames along the length of the device implanted
Scaffold area		At baseline, the scaffold area is measured by joining the middle points of the abluminal sides of the black cores of the apposed struts or the abluminal edge of the frame borders of malapposed struts. At follow-up, the abluminal side of the central black core is used to delimit the scaffold area
Blood flow area	(Scaffold area + ISA area) − (intraluminal strut areas + prolapse area + intraluminal defect area)	
Neointimal hyperplasia area	i. In case of all struts apposed Scaffold area − [lumen area + black box area] ii. In case of malapposed struts [Scaffold area + ISA area + malapposed strut with surrounding tissues] − [lumen area + strut area]	Note the difference of methodology with that of gray-scale IVUS
Thickness of tissue coverage	Distance between the abluminal site of the strut and the lumen − strut thickness	Since the strut thickness is 150 μm (ABSORB), the strut was considered as covered whenever the thickness of the coverage was more than this threshold value. This method may slightly underestimate the thickness of the coverage because it does not take into account changes in the size of the strut core over time

Adapted from Garcia-Garcia HM, Serruys PW, Campos CM, et al. Assessing bioresorbable coronary devices: methods and parameters. JACC Cardiovasc Imaging 2014;7:1130–48.

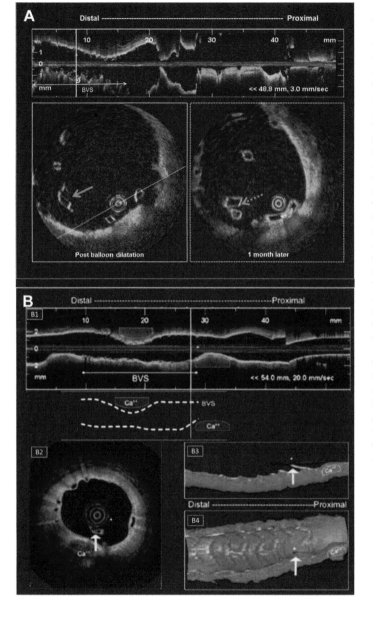

Fig. 3. Representative OCT image of scaffold fracture and discontinuity. (A) Scaffold fracture. During the index procedure after postdilatation of an Absorb BVS, OCT cross-sectional image shows scaffold fracture (*blue arrow, left*). The strut luminal and abluminal surfaces are no longer orientated perpendicular to the light source. OCT cross-sectional image 1 month later shows extensive strut disarray (*dotted blue arrow, right*). (B) Scaffold discontinuity. OCT acquisition 6 months after Absorb BVS implantation. In the 2-dimensional (cross-sectional) OCT image, extreme malapposition of 1 strut is seen (panel *B2, yellow arrow*). In the 3-dimensional reconstruction, the overhanging strut is clearly identified in its whole trajectory (panel *B3, B4; yellow arrow*). Further intervention was deferred because of lack of ischemic symptoms. ([A] *Adapted from* Ormiston JA, De Vroey F, Serruys PW, et al. Bioresorbable polymeric vascular scaffolds: a cautionary tale. Circ Cardiovasc Interv 2011;4:535–8; and [B] *From* Garcia-Garcia HM, Serruys PW, Campos CM, et al. Assessing bioresorbable coronary devices: methods and parameters. JACC Cardiovasc Imaging 2014;7:1130–48.)

have resolved. In serial OCT analysis of BRSs, postprocedural proximal edge dissection was noted in 21% of cases and distal edge dissection in 38% of cases, compared with 2% and 5% at 6 months, respectively. At 1 year, an edge dissection was present in only 2% (proximal) and none were observed at 2- and 3-year follow-up. No scaffold thrombosis was reported in this trial.[8] Therefore, although edge dissection by OCT is often detected, most of these dissections healed within 6 months without any clinical sequelae. However, the small sample size of this study limits any definitive conclusion with respect to the effect of residual edge dissection on clinical outcomes.

Eccentricity and Symmetry

The eccentricity and symmetry of implanted BRSs are easily assessed by OCT (see Table 2). These parameters have been shown to be associated with clinical outcomes after metallic stents.[9,10] With the clinical adoption of various

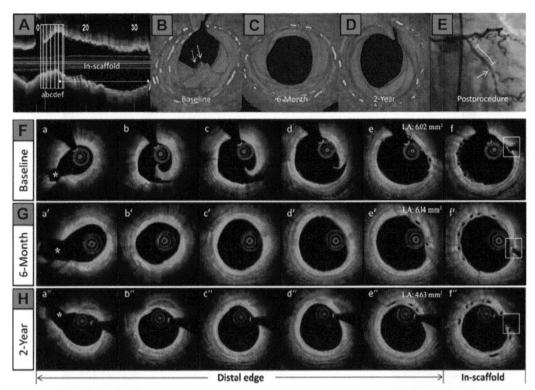

Fig. 4. Representative imaging of a dissection at the distal edge of Absorb BVS. (A) Longitudinal view of a distal dissection. (B) Three-dimensional reconstruction of OCT pullback showing luminal disruption at distal edge of the scaffold (*double white arrow*). (C, D) Three-dimensional reconstruction at 6-month and 2-year follow-up, respectively, demonstrating that the dissection has healed. (E) No distal edge dissection is visible from the angiograms postprocedure (*yellow arrow*). (F) OCT cross-sectional images immediately after implantation show that a dissection extends into the media. (G) OCT image at 6-month follow-up demonstrates an increase in lumen area at that region without visible dissection. (H) At 2-year follow-up, the lumen area has decreased with detected calcific tissue. *Asterisk*, side branch. (*From* Zhang YJ, Iqbal J, Nakatani S, et al. ABSORB Cohort B Study Investigators. Scaffold and edge vascular response following implantation of everolimus-eluting bioresorbable vascular scaffold: a 3 year serial optical coherence tomography study. JACC Cardiovasc Interv 2014;7(12):1361–9.)

bioresorbable devices, the reevaluation of the clinical effect of these geometric parameters is required at short- and long-term follow-up. The eccentricity ratio is defined as the ratio of the minimum and maximum diameters of the scaffold in each frame. The eccentricity index is obtained by calculating the average of all eccentricity ratios along the length of the scaffold.[3] The symmetry index is derived from the maximum scaffold diameter and minimum scaffold diameter along the length of the BRS, which may be located within different frames. It is calculated as the difference between the maximum scaffold diameter and the minimum scaffold diameter, divided by the maximum scaffold diameter.[3] It must be emphasized that the maximum and the minimum scaffold diameters

in this calculation may be located in 2 different frames along the length of the implanted device (Fig. 5).

Bioresorbable Scaffold Versus Drug-Eluting Stent at Time of Implantation

BRSs have distinct mechanical properties compared with metallic stents that could influence the aforementioned OCT parameters. Mattesini and colleagues[11] compared the final, postimplantation results of the Absorb BVS and second-generation drug-eluting stents (DESs) using OCT. A total of 50 complex coronary lesions (class B2/C by the American College of Cardiology/American Heart Association definition) treated with a BVS undergoing a final OCT examination were compared with an equal

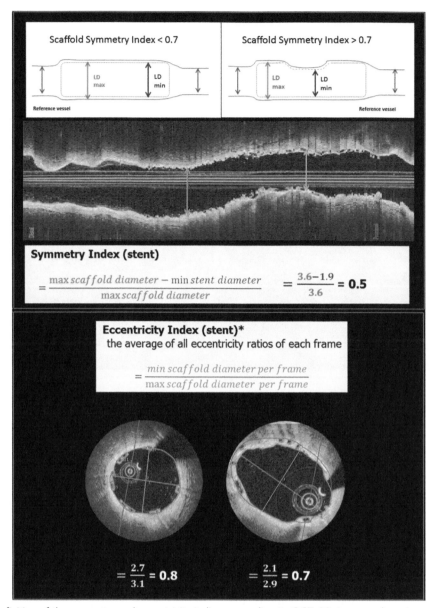

Fig. 5. Definition of the symmetry and eccentricity indices according to OCT. Minimum and maximum diameters along the length of the device are shown. Two cross-sections with different eccentricity indices are also shown.

number of matched lesions treated with second-generation DESs. In the BRS group, there was more extensive lesion preparation (eg, significantly greater balloon diameter:reference vessel diameter ratio and higher inflation predilation pressure) and significantly higher postdilatation pressure used. Final OCT examination demonstrated a trend toward greater tissue prolapse area ($P = .08$) and a significantly higher rate of proximal edge ISA ($P = .04$) in the BVS group. There was no significant difference in the overall ISA, mean lumen area, and eccentricity index between the 2 groups. There were 2 cases of strut fractures in the lesions treated with BVS, whereas none was observed with DES.[11]

OPTICAL COHERENCE TOMOGRAPHIC EVALUATION OF BIORESORBABLE SCAFFOLD OVER LONG-TERM FOLLOW-UP

Because BRSs are designed to degrade with time after implantation, the structural characteristics of the scaffold are dynamic and can be well visualized by OCT imaging. Key parameters that may be assessed during ongoing follow-up include the presence of any scaffold discontinuity, scaffold eccentricity, strut coverage, and neointimal hyperplasia.

Scaffold Discontinuity

OCT may detect scaffold discontinuity during the process of resorption. The assessment of scaffold discontinuity is the same as that of scaffold fracture after short-term BRS implantation, that is, discontinuity is present if 2 struts overhang each other in the same angular sector of the lumen perimeter, with or without malapposition, or if isolated struts are located near the center of the vessel lumen without obvious connection with other surrounding struts in the 2-dimensional image. Three-dimensional OCT reconstruction is helpful to better understand scaffold discontinuity (see Fig. 3B).

Eccentricity

As the scaffold degrades, its biomechanical properties are altered, and therefore, eccentricity may change with time and should be assessed for new BRSs. In a small series of 8 patients with 5-year follow-up after Absorb BVS implantation, eccentricity decreased with time (see Fig. 5, Table 2).[12]

Strut Coverage and Neointimal Hyperplasia

The analysis of strut coverage is complex, as it must take into account the embedding and thickening of the frame borders, along with a reduction of the strut central core. The strut area is defined only by its black core, because the light-scattering frame is no longer distinguishable from the surrounding tissue and the tissue begins to fill the strut area, a phenomenon that can be identified by irregular, high-intensity areas. At follow-up, the luminal area follows the endoluminal contour of the neointima between and on top of the apposed struts; this can be traced by semiautomatic detection. In the case of malapposed struts, the endoluminal contour of the vessel wall behind the malapposed struts should be used to define the luminal border. The abluminal side of the central black core is used to delimit the scaffold area. If all struts are apposed, neointimal hyperplasia area is calculated as the difference between the scaffold area and the sum of the lumen and black box areas (ie, scaffold area − [lumen area + black box area]). In the setting of malapposed struts, neointimal hyperplasia area is calculated by subtracting the sum of the lumen and strut areas from the sum of the scaffold area, ISA area, and the area of malapposed struts and

surrounding tissues (ie, [scaffold area + ISA area + malapposed strut with surrounding tissues] − [lumen area + strut area]) (see Fig. 2C, Table 2).

SERIAL OPTICAL COHERENCE TOMOGRAPHIC OBSERVATIONS IN SCAFFOLDED SEGMENTS

The OCT results of Absorb BVS Cohorts B1 and B2 have been reported up to 3-year follow-up. The findings of these OCT analyses are illustrated in Fig. 6. There was an initial decrease

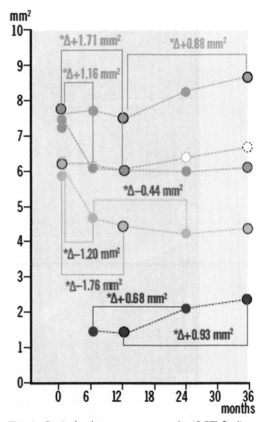

Fig. 6. Optical coherence tomography (OCT) findings in ABSORB Cohort B trial. OCT was performed postprocedure, at 6, 12, 24, and 36 months. The different parameters are color coded. ●, Scaffold area in cohort B1; ○, scaffold area in cohort B2; ●, mean lumen area in cohort B1; ○, mean lumen area in cohort B2; , minimum scaffold area in cohort B1; ○, Minimum scaffold area in cohort B2; ●, minimum lumen area in cohort B1; ○, minimum lumen area in cohort B2; ●, neointimal area in cohort B1; ●, neointimal area in cohort B2. (*Adapted from* Serruys PW, Onuma Y, Garcia-Garcia HM, et al. Dynamics of vessel wall changes following the implantation of the absorb everolimus-eluting bioresorbable vascular scaffold: a multi-imaging modality study at 6, 12, 24 and 36 months. EuroIntervention 2014;9(11):1271–84.)

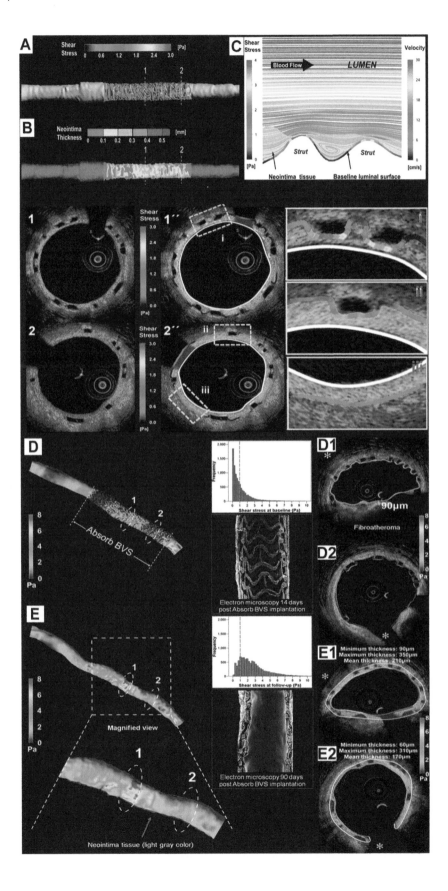

in the minimal and mean lumen area that stabilized over the longer term. Although there was an increase in neointima between 1 and 3 years, it was compensated by the parallel increase in the mean and minimum scaffold area, thereby maintaining the lumen area unchanged. A total of 98% percent of struts were covered, and 3 of the 13 scaffolds had malapposed struts with an average malapposition area of 0.60 mm^2.[13] Serial OCT evaluation of edge and scaffold vascular responses of the Absorb BVS showed less lumen loss at the edges than lumen loss within the scaffold.[8] Neointimal coverage of the Absorb BVS seems to be driven by shear stress patterns of the blood flow (Fig. 7).

Serial OCT examinations have demonstrated that Absorb BVS may potentially passivate vulnerable plaques (Fig. 8).[14] In one such study, 46 patients treated with Absorb BVS and 20 patients treated with bare metal stents (Svelte coronary Integrated Delivery System, a balloon-expandable, cobalt-chromium, thin-strut fixed wire stent) had thin-capped fibroatheromas (TCFAs) identified within the device implantation regions and in the adjacent native coronary segments. At 6- to 12-month follow-up, only 8% of the TCFAs detected at baseline were still present within the Absorb BVS compared with 27% within the bare metal stent implantation segments ($P = .231$). A total of 60% of the TCFAs in native segments did not change their phenotype at follow-up. The more aggressive neointimal response to the bare metal stent resulted in a greater reduction in luminal dimensions compared with the Absorb BVS. The loss of the scaffold's structural integrity allowed the device to expand and accommodate the tissue that developed and recapped the underlying high-risk plaques.[14]

The serial changes in atherosclerotic plaques after BRS implantation can be quantified by OCT. In ex vivo validation studies, highly attenuating regions (attenuation coefficient $\mu t \geq 8$ mm^{-1}) seen on OCT have been associated with the presence of necrotic core or macrophages. Conversely, attenuation coefficient less than 6 mm^{-1} was associated with healthy vessels, calcified plaque, or intimal thickening.[15,16] In a small series of 8 patients with 5-year follow-up after Absorb BVS implantation, OCT demonstrated a low-attenuating layer covering the treated atherosclerotic plaques (Fig. 9). In 1 patient, a TCFA was observed at

Fig. 7. (A–C) Distribution of the endothelial shear stress (ESS) and neointimal thickness (NT) in a scaffolded segment. The dashed lines in the reconstructed segment in (A) and (B) indicate the location of the optical coherence tomographic images in 1 and 2. 1″ and 2″ show the ESS distribution across the circumference of the vessel wall; the neointimal thickness is portrayed in a semitransparent manner. As shown in i, ii, and iii, the ESS is low in the between-strut areas and high on top of the struts. The neointimal tissue appears to be increased in segments with low ESS and reduced in segments with high ESS values. The blood flow streamlines are shown with velocity color coding (right), whereas the ESS distribution along the baseline luminal surface is portrayed according to the color-coded map (left). The neointimal thickness at 1-year follow-up is shown in a semitransparent fashion. Low ESS and recirculation zones are noted in the interstrut areas, whereas ESS values are high on top of the struts. The ESS distribution seems to affect neointimal formation, because there is increased neointimal tissue in the regions between the struts and minimal neointimal tissue over the struts. (D) Three-dimensional reconstruction of coronary anatomy from the baseline coronary angiographic and OCT data and blood flow simulation, with the local ESS being portrayed in a color-coded map (blue indicates low ESS and red, high ESS). The distribution of the ESS in the scaffolded segment is illustrated at the top right side of the panel, whereas below there is an electron microscopic image acquired 14 days after Absorb BVS implantation in an animal model showing the rugged luminal surface. (D1, D2) Baseline ESS distribution around the circumference of the vessel wall in 2 OCT cross-sectional images. Normal to high ESS noted over a fibroatheroma with a cap thickness of 90 mm in D1, whereas in D2, the ESS is low over the vessel wall and normal over the struts. The asterisk in both images indicates a side branch. At follow-up, the ESS values are normalized in the scaffolded segment and seem to be increased when compared with baseline (E). The magnified view demonstrates the thin layer of neointima that has developed and is portrayed with light gray. High ESS was noted over the fibroatheroma detected at baseline, but the neointimal tissue has sealed the plaque (E1). The low ESS estimated at baseline across the circumference of the vessel wall in D2 is normalized at follow-up (E2). ([A–C] Adapted from Bourantas CV, Papafaklis MI, Kotsia A, et al. Effect of the endothelial shear stress patterns on neointimal proliferation following drug-eluting bioresorbable vascular scaffold implantation: an optical coherence tomography study. JACC Cardiovasc Interv 2014;7:315–24; and [D, E] From Bourantas CV, Papafaklis MI, Garcia-Garcia HM, et al. Short- and long-term implications of a bioresorbable vascular scaffold implantation on the local endothelial shear stress patterns. JACC Cardiovasc Interv 2014;7:100–1.)

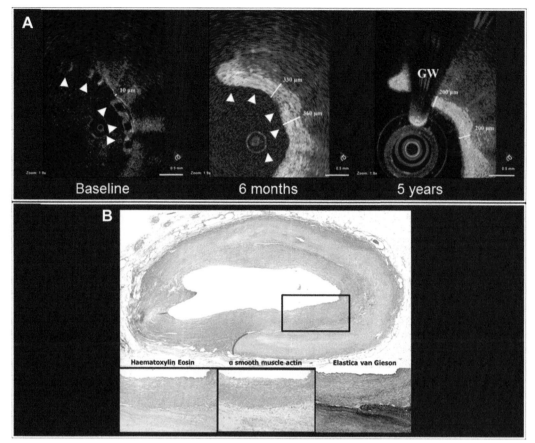

Fig. 8. (A) OCT images acquired from a matched site at baseline, 6 months, and 5 years after Absorb BVS implantation. The amount of tissue overlying the calcific deposition increased from baseline to 6 months because of neointimal response to scaffold implantation. At 5 years, the scaffold struts and neointima have merged into a thick layer of tissue covering the underlying plaque. Arrowheads indicate scaffold struts. GW indicates guidewire artifact. (B) Histologic findings 10 years after Igaki-Tamai bioresorbable scaffold implantation at the left anterior descending coronary artery. The spaces previously occupied by PLLA scaffold struts disappeared. Elastica van Gieson staining shows thick intima. This thick intima consisted of smooth muscle cells and fibrotic tissues without almost no inflammatory cells. ([A] *Adapted from* Karanasos A, Simsek C, Gnanadesigan M, et al. OCT assessment of the long-term vascular healing response 5 years after everolimus-eluting bioresorbable vascular scaffold. J Am Coll Cardiol 2014;64(22):2343–56.)

the distal scaffold segment with cap disruption and small thrombus.[16] Qualitatively, comparison with prior follow-up OCT examinations did not demonstrate any evidence for the accumulation of de novo adluminal necrotic core within the scaffolded segments.[16] Conversely, patients treated with metallic DESs seemed to develop neoatherosclerosis within the neointima (see Fig. 9).[16] Given the small sample size, and the observation of a different tissue response in 1 patient, these findings require confirmation in larger studies.

OPTICAL COHERENCE TOMOGRAPHY AND SCAFFOLD DEGRADATION

OCT may not be sensitive enough to assess the extent of polymer degradation. The absence of strut footprints on OCT was at first interpreted as a sign of complete bioresorption; however, it was subsequently shown that OCT cannot differentiate the polylactide of the polymer from the provisional matrix of proteoglycan formed by connective tissue.[13,17] Thus, polymer may no longer be present in the black core areas

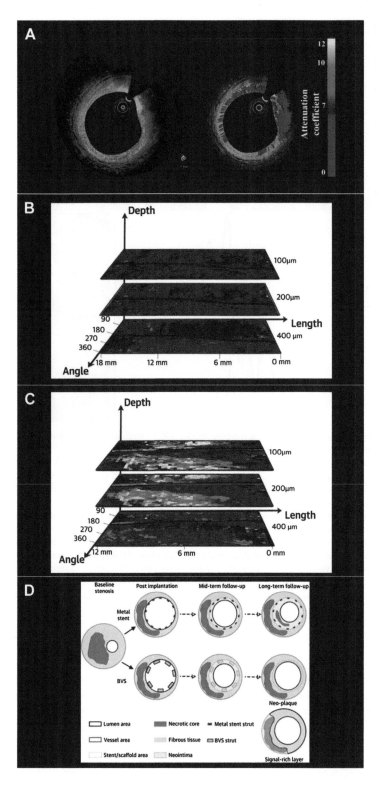

Fig. 9. (A) Example of attenuation analysis. Tissue attenuation properties within adluminal and abluminal contour are measured in all frames and displayed on a color scale (blue represents low-attenuation regions, whereas red and yellow represent high-attenuation regions). For intimal thickness less than 200 mm, as in the 6-o'clock to 7-o'clock position, analysis is not performed because of lack of a sufficient imaging window. (B, C) Spread-out maps demonstrating attenuation coefficient in predefined depths from the vessel surface (100, 200, and 400 mm). In (B) there is a low-attenuating layer of 200 mm separating the underlying plaque (starting at ~400 μm) from the lumen. In (C), this layer was absent, and attenuating areas were close to the lumen. (D) Potential paradigm shift in the treatment of atherosclerosis with Absorb BVS. After metal stent implantation, struts are preserved and the neointimal area clearly delineated between stent and lumen contour even at long-term follow-up. There is a possible development of neoatherosclerosis within the neointima. Conversely, bioresorbable scaffolds in long-term follow-up of the neointimal boundaries are unclear after degradation (dotted line), and the intima resembles native plaque, defined as neoplaque. The signal-rich layer is the layer that separates the underlying plaque components from the lumen. (Adapted from Karanasos A, Simsek C, Gnanadesigan M, et al. OCT assessment of the long-term vascular healing response 5 years after everolimus-eluting bioresorbable vascular scaffold. J Am Coll Cardiol 2014;64(22):2343–56.)

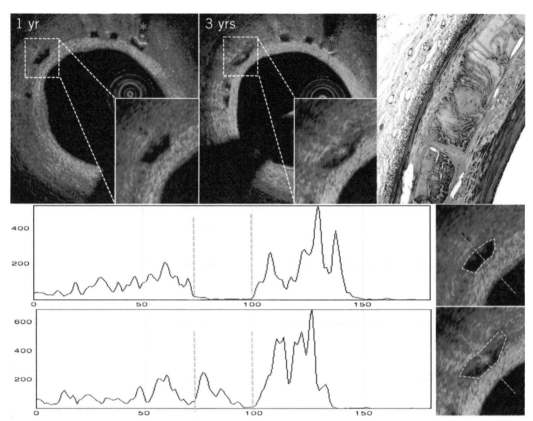

Fig. 10. Comparison of serial OCT and histologic findings in a porcine model. OCT cross sections were matched according to the presence of distal metallic markers (*red asterisks*) at 1 and 3 years. One of the matched struts next to the marker (*asterisk*) was analyzed by light reflectivity.[21] At 3 years, the strut core that was initially black became partially filled by a nucleus exhibiting high light reflectivity. Tracings at the bottom showed graphically the light reflectivity along the scan line of incident light (*red*). The vertical green dotted lines correspond to the adluminal and abluminal boundaries of the black core either empty or partially occupied by white nucleus. Histologic picture (Movat staining) of porcine coronary artery 36 months after implantation of Absorb scaffold showed provisional matrix (glycoconjugates) in purple, filling the void previously occupied by the polymeric strut. A cellularized (*black dots*) area with connective tissue (*green staining*) is located at the center of the strut void and is connected to the subintima. Multilayers of smooth muscle cells are overlying the strut voids. OCT images of the histologic structures in a porcine model are similar to those observed in human. (*Adapted from* Serruys PW, Onuma Y, Garcia-Garcia HM, et al. Dynamics of vessel wall changes following the implantation of the Absorb everolimus-eluting bioresorbable vascular scaffold: a multi-imaging modality study at 6, 12, 24 and 36 months. EuroIntervention 2014;9(11):1271–84.)

seen on OCT. OCT does provide information regarding scaffold integration, that is, when the scaffold struts start to have cellular areas with connective tissue (**Fig. 10**).[13,17]

OVERLAPPING SEGMENTS, BIFURCATIONS, AND 2-DIMENSIONAL VERSUS 3-DIMENSIONAL OPTICAL COHERENCE TOMOGRAPHY

Three-dimensional OCT provides much more useful information at bifurcations and overlapping segments than does 2-dimensional OCT. In overlapping regions, 2-dimensional OCT helps to identify single or stacked struts (inner vs outer) and stacked strut clusters (**Fig. 11**). Lumen area should be calculated similarly to nonoverlapping segments. Scaffold area at overlapping segments should be calculated by planimetry from the backside (ie, abluminal side) of the black core area of the outermost strut or stacked strut cluster (at the point of all the struts apposing the vessel endothelium) apposing the vessel wall. Where there does not

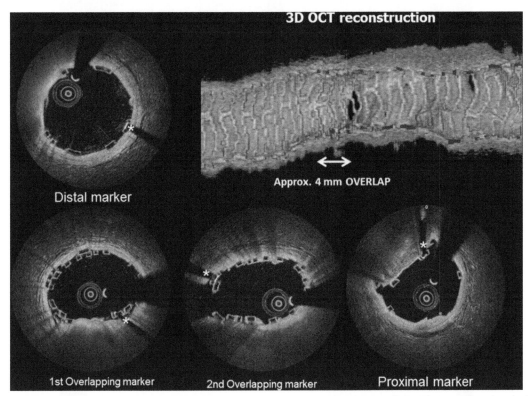

Fig. 11. In the cross-sectional images of optical coherence tomography, the metallic markers can be identified as high-echogenic and high–light intensity structures accompanied with backward shadows (*asterisks*). The 3-dimensional OCT reconstruction helps to understand the overlapping region. (*From* Garcia-Garcia HM, Serruys PW, Campos CM, et al. Assessing bioresorbable coronary devices: methods and parameters. JACC Cardiovasc Imaging 2014;7:1130–48.)

appear to be any apposition of a single strut or stacked strut cluster to the vessel endothelium, the contour of the scaffold area continues to follow the outermost (most abluminal) scaffold strut or stacked strut cluster. Three-dimensional OCT of overlapping regions helps define the type of overlapping, interdigitating struts versus complete overlap.[18]

Within bifurcations, 3-dimensional OCT enables a detailed assessment of both the longitudinal and cross-sectional relationship between the jailed side branch orifice and the overhanging struts.[19] Modifications of the shape of the struts after side branch dilatation can be observed with 3-dimensional OCT. Serial 3-dimensional OCT provides information regarding the evolution of the bifurcation anatomy after scaffold implantation, such as the presence of neointimal bridges, which usually appear as an extension of the preexisting carina. From a quantitative point of view, 3-dimensional OCT reconstruction can be used to assess the changes over time in the number of compartments and their geometric areas (Fig. 12).

AGREEMENT AND REPRODUCIBILITY OF OPTICAL COHERENCE TOMOGRAPHY FOR THE ASSESSMENT OF BIORESORBABLE SCAFFOLDS

OCT has excellent reproducibility for the assessment of incomplete malapposition and struts at side branches.[20] OCT is the most accurate technique for measuring scaffold length. There is a moderate agreement with IVUS in the measurement of in-scaffold minimum lumen area assessment at the same coronary segment, and therefore their values should not be used interchangeably.[5]

348

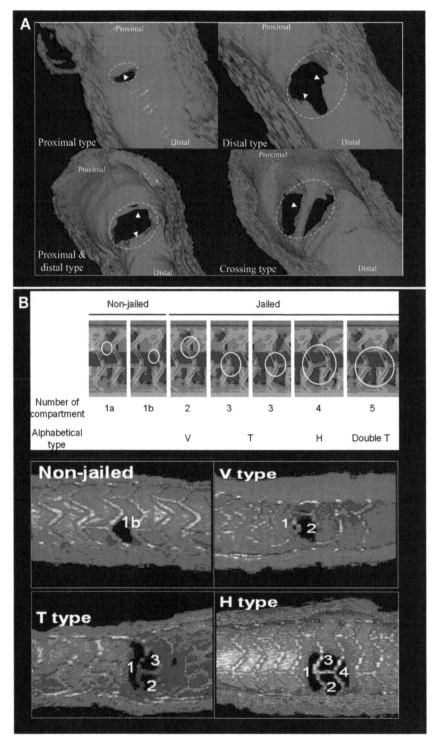

Fig. 12. Three-dimensional OCT side branch classification. (A) Classification based on the relative location with the side-branch ostium. Four different types could be identified: proximal, distal, proximal and distal, or crossing. Dotted lines indicate side-branch ostia; arrowheads indicate tissue bridge. (B) Upper panel shows the bioresorbable vascular scaffold (BVS) with polymeric struts. Yellow circles represent the orifice of the side branch (SB). A nonjailed SB is defined as the complete absence of struts across the orifice (1a) or BVS struts located over the orifice without compartmentalization (1b). Lower panel shows jailed SB orifices are separated into various compartments. Types of SB jailing are expressed in alphabetical letters given according to resemblance of the strut structure across the orifice. ([A] From Karanasos A, Simsek C, Gnanadesigan M, et al. OCT assessment of the long-term vascular healing response 5 years after everolimus-eluting bioresorbable vascular scaffold. J Am Coll Cardiol 2014;64(22):2343–56; and [B] Adapted from Okamura T, Onuma Y, Garcia-Garcia HM, et al. 3-Dimensional optical coherence tomography assessment of jailed side branches by bioresorbable vascular scaffolds: a proposal for classification. JACC Cardiovasc Interv 2010;3:836–44.)

SUMMARY

OCT is a valuable tool for BRS assessment because of its high resolution. It provides detailed and reproducible information regarding the interaction between the device and lumen surface. A dedicated methodology for OCT analysis, different from that for metallic stents, is required for the short- and long-term assessment of BRS.

REFERENCES

1. Serruys PW, Garcia-Garcia HM, Onuma Y. From metallic cages to transient bioresorbable scaffolds: change in paradigm of coronary revascularization in the upcoming decade? Eur Heart J 2012;33:16–25b.
2. Waksman R. Biodegradable stents: they do their job and disappear. J Invasive Cardiol 2006;18:70–4.
3. Garcia-Garcia HM, Serruys PW, Campos CM, et al. Assessing bioresorbable coronary devices: methods and parameters. JACC Cardiovasc Imaging 2014;7:1130–48.
4. Campos CM, Lemos PA. Bioresorbable vascular scaffolds: novel devices, novel interpretations, and novel interventions strategies. Catheter Cardiovasc Interv 2014;84:46–7.
5. Gutierrez-Chico JL, Serruys PW, Girasis C, et al. Quantitative multi-modality imaging analysis of a fully bioresorbable stent: a head-to-head comparison between QCA, IVUS and OCT. Int J Cardiovasc Imaging 2012;28:467–78.
6. Gutierrez H, Arnold R, Gimeno F, et al. Optical coherence tomography. Initial experience in patients undergoing percutaneous coronary intervention. Rev Esp Cardiol 2008;61:976–9.
7. Radu MD, Raber L, Heo J, et al. Natural history of optical coherence tomography-detected non-flow-limiting edge dissections following drug-eluting stent implantation. EuroIntervention 2014;9:1085–94.
8. Zhang YJ, Iqbal J, Nakatani S, et al, ABSORB Cohort B Study Investigators. Scaffold and edge vascular response following implantation of everolimus-eluting bioresorbable vascular scaffold: a 3 year serial optical coherence tomography study. JACC Cardiovasc Interv 2014;7(12):1361–9.
9. de Jaegere P, Mudra H, Figulla H, et al. Intravascular ultrasound-guided optimized stent deployment. Immediate and 6 months clinical and angiographic results from the Multicenter Ultrasound Stenting in Coronaries Study (MUSIC Study). Eur Heart J 1998;19:1214–23.
10. Otake H, Shite J, Ako J, et al. Local determinants of thrombus formation following sirolimus-eluting stent implantation assessed by optical coherence tomography. JACC Cardiovasc Interv 2009;2:459–66.
11. Mattesini A, Secco GG, Dall'Ara G, et al. ABSORB biodegradable stents versus second-generation metal stents: a comparison study of 100 complex lesions treated under OCT guidance. JACC Cardiovasc Interv 2014;7:741–50.
12. Karanasos A, Simsek C, Gnanadesigan M, et al. OCT assessment of the long-term vascular healing response 5 years after everolimus-eluting bioresorbable vascular scaffold. J Am Coll Cardiol 2014;64(22):2343–56.
13. Serruys PW, Onuma Y, Garcia-Garcia HM, et al. Dynamics of vessel wall changes following the implantation of the Absorb everolimus-eluting bioresorbable vascular scaffold: a multi-imaging modality study at 6, 12, 24 and 36 months. EuroIntervention 2014;9(11):1271–84.
14. Bourantas CV, Serruys PW, Nakatani S, et al. Bioresorbable vascular scaffold treatment induces the formation of neointimal cap that seals the underlying plaque without compromising the luminal dimensions: a concept based on serial optical coherence tomography data. EuroIntervention 2014. [Epub ahead of print].
15. van Soest G, Goderie T, Regar E, et al. Atherosclerotic tissue characterization in vivo by optical coherence tomography attenuation imaging. J Biomed Opt 2010;15:011105.
16. Ughi GJ, Adriaenssens T, Sinnaeve P, et al. Automated tissue characterization of in vivo atherosclerotic plaques by intravascular optical coherence tomography images. Biomed Opt Express 2013;4:1014–30.
17. Onuma Y, Serruys PW, Perkins LE, et al. Intracoronary optical coherence tomography and histology at 1 month and 2, 3, and 4 years after implantation of everolimus-eluting bioresorbable vascular scaffolds in a porcine coronary artery model: an attempt to decipher the human optical coherence tomography images in the ABSORB trial. Circulation 2010;122:2288–300.
18. Farooq V, Onuma Y, Radu M, et al. Optical coherence tomography (OCT) of overlapping bioresorbable scaffolds: from benchwork to clinical application. EuroIntervention 2011;7:386–99.
19. Okamura T, Onuma Y, Garcia-Garcia HM, et al. 3-Dimensional optical coherence tomography assessment of jailed side branches by bioresorbable vascular scaffolds: a proposal for classification. JACC Cardiovasc Interv 2010;3:836–44.
20. Gomez-Lara J, Brugaletta S, Diletti R, et al. Agreement and reproducibility of gray-scale intravascular ultrasound and optical coherence tomography for the analysis of the bioresorbable vascular scaffold. Catheter Cardiovasc Interv 2012;79:890–902.
21. Nakatani S, Onuma Y, Ishibashi Y, et al. Temporal evolution of strut light intensity after implantation of bioresorbable polymeric intracoronary scaffolds in the ABSORB Cohort B trial - an application of a new quantitative method based on optical coherence tomography. Circ J 2014;78:1873–81.

Advances in Automated Assessment of Intracoronary Optical Coherence Tomography and Their Clinical Application

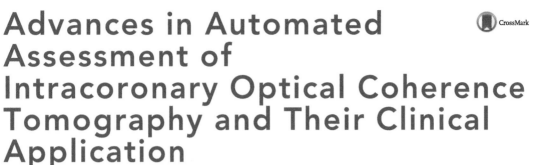

Giovanni J. Ughi, PhD[a,b],
Tom Adriaenssens, MD, PhD[a,b,c,*]

KEYWORDS

- Optical coherence tomography • OCT • Intravascular imaging • Image processing
- Automated image analysis • Stent • Atherosclerosis

KEY POINTS

- Intravascular optical coherence tomography (OCT) is capable of acquiring 3-dimensional (3D) data of coronary arteries allowing for the assessment of plaques, stents, thrombus, side branches, and other relevant structures in a 3D fashion.
- Given that state-of-the-art OCT systems acquire images at a very high frame rate (up to 200 frames per second), typically a very large number of images per pullback (ie, 500 or more) need to be analyzed.
- The manual assessment of stents, plaques, and other structures is time-consuming, cumbersome, and inefficient and thus not suitable for on-line analysis during percutaneous coronary intervention procedures; similarly, manual analysis is also inefficient in the setting of preclinical studies and clinical trials.

INTRODUCTION

Intravascular optical coherence tomography (OCT) is a high-resolution imaging technique using a near-infrared laser source (wavelength of ~1310 nm) and interferometry acquiring images of vessel wall microstructure and morphology.[1] State-of-the-art OCT has an axial resolution less than 15 μm and a lateral resolution ~30 to 60 μm, and it shows a penetration depth up to 3 mm in the coronary artery wall.[2] If compared with other imaging techniques, such as intravascular ultrasound (IVUS), computed tomographic

scan, MRI, and MR angiography, it provides orders of magnitudes improvement in terms of image resolution.[3] Similarly to IVUS, OCT is an invasive catheter-based imaging technique, capable of acquiring multiple cross-sectional images of long segments of coronary arteries (typically 5–10 cm) in a few seconds, using a contrast injection to get the vessel lumen cleared from blood.

OCT is extensively used for the assessment of intravascular devices (i.e., intracoronary stents) and for the assessment of human atherosclerosis in vivo.[4,5] It allows quantification of both acute

The authors have nothing to disclose.
[a] Department of Cardiovascular Sciences, Katholieke Universiteit Leuven, Herestraat 49, 3000 Leuven, Belgium;
[b] Department of Cardiovascular Diseases, University Hospitals Leuven, Herestraat 49, 3000 Leuven, Belgium;
[c] Department of Cardiovascular Medicine, University Hospitals Leuven, Herestraat 49, 3000 Leuven, Belgium
* Corresponding author. Department of Cardiology, University Hospitals Leuven, Herestraat 49, 3000 Leuven, Belgium.
E-mail address: tom.adriaenssens@uzleuven.be

and late stent strut apposition to the vessel wall, the latter of which has been correlated with late stent failure.[6] Similarly, it allows assessment of the lack of stent strut neointimal coverage, a predictor of stent thrombosis.[7] OCT is able to discriminate stable plaques (e.g., fibrotic or calcific) from high-risk thin-cap fibroatheromas (lipid/necrotic core).[5] Moreover, OCT acquires 3-dimensional (3D) data of coronary arteries, allowing for the assessment of plaques, stents, thrombus, side branches, and other relevant structures in a 3D fashion.[8] As such, OCT is extensively used in assessing the safety and efficacy of novel therapies and interventions for the management of stable coronary artery disease and acute coronary syndromes as well as for the optimization of percutaneous coronary interventions (PCI).[9,10]

Given that state-of-the-art OCT systems acquire images at a very high frame rate (up to 200 frames per second), typically a very large number of cross-sectional images per pullback (ie, 500 or more) need to be analyzed. As such, manual analysis is very time-consuming, making the manual assessment of stents, plaques, and other structures very cumbersome and inefficient and thus not suitable for on-line analysis during PCI. Similarly, manual analysis is also very inefficient for clinical/preclinical studies and trials, where typically a very high number of images need to be analyzed.

This article focuses on currently available automated methods for the analysis of OCT datasets and discusses future directions and current needs of the OCT community.

METHODS FOR AUTOMATED INTRAVASCULAR OPTICAL COHERENCE TOMOGRAPHY IMAGE ANALYSIS

Several methods and software prototypes to analyze OCT data, with many different aims and objectives, have been developed over the past few years. These methods and software prototypes can be broadly divided into 4 different groups: (1) automated assessment of lumen morphology; (2) automated analysis of stents; (3) automated plaque analysis and tissue characterization; and (4) advanced methods for the analysis of other structures and OCT image features (eg, macrophages and thrombus).

Although some software prototypes are currently available for research purposes, currently there is neither standardization nor a common validation dataset for the different methods. Efforts from the OCT community will be required to define a standard for the validation and use of the recently proposed methods.

Automated Assessment of Lumen Morphology

OCT allows for the visualization of vessel morphology with great detail. One of the most direct and useful applications of OCT is the automated assessment of lumen contour, quantifying minimal cross-sectional area (eg, lumen narrowing), the extension of the lesion and reference (i.e., normal) vessel diameter in a 3D fashion through an entire OCT pullback (Fig. 1).

For this purpose, many different approaches have been developed, typically showing a very high correlation with respect to the gold standard (i.e., manual analysis).[11,12] These different approaches are currently available on commercial OCT systems (St. Jude Medical, St. Paul, MN, USA; and Terumo Corporation, Tokyo, Japan).[13] Such strategies typically segment the lumen contour through an entire intravascular OCT dataset in an automated fashion, eventually allowing the user to manually correct segmentation results in case of artifact or challenging situations. These methods are typically based on the gray-scale analysis of OCT images taking advantage of vessel spatial continuity to achieve a robust segmentation of the vessel wall.

Such algorithms typically allow for a reliable 2-dimensional (2D)/3D representation of vessel area complementing angiography during PCI and may be of help for the identification and characterization of the culprit lesion (e.g., plaque extension) as well as for a better assessment of in-stent restenosis. Moreover, the segmentation of vessel lumen is not only a useful tool to automatically quantify vessel area but also one of the basic features for more advanced processing algorithms that aim to automatically quantify stent strut apposition/coverage as well as perform tissue characterization and automated 3D renderings.

Automated Stent Analysis

Among the many applications of intravascular OCT, its use for the quantitative assessment of stent strut apposition and coverage is one of the most important. Given that persistent stent strut malapposition and lack of neointimal coverage have been correlated with adverse events (e.g., late stent thrombosis), OCT findings have been used extensively as a surrogate marker for the safety and efficacy profile of coronary stents. Manual analysis of stents by OCT must quantify the amount of malapposed struts, the severity of malapposition, and the amount of struts not showing sufficient neointimal coverage (i.e., lack of coverage) (Fig. 2). This kind of analysis requires manual detection and

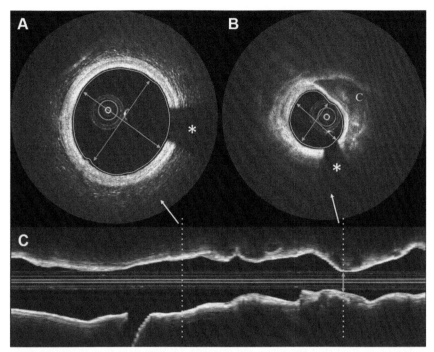

Fig. 1. Quantification of lumen morphology (lumen area, maximum and minimum diameters). (*A*) Cross-sectional image of a normal segment of a coronary artery not showing any narrowing. (*B*) Partial but severe lumen narrowing (minimal lumen area) due to a calcified plaque. (*C*) A longitudinal view of the entire vessel, where the minimal luminal area is clearly visible. Automatic segmentation and quantification of lumen morphology allow for a complete assessment of luminal narrowing, helping in the assessment of lesion extension. The asterisk (*) indicates the guidewire shadowing artifact. C, calcified plaque.

measurement of each strut location with respect to the lumen contour, resulting in a very labor-intensive procedure. Given that intravascular OCT pullbacks contain hundreds of frames, this kind of analysis can be extremely time-consuming (several hours for a detailed analysis), making it impractical not only for on-line OCT image analysis but also for preclinical and clinical studies and trials. As such, algorithms for the automatic segmentation of stent struts[11,12,14,15] and thus the automatic quantification of malapposition and neointimal coverage[11,16] are extremely important to achieve an efficient analysis. These approaches have been shown to significantly speed up the analysis of OCT datasets. Moreover, novel methods for the automatic quantification of malapposed/uncovered stent struts 3D distribution were recently shown to achieve a more complete OCT analysis of intracoronary stents with respect to the standard manual analysis (ie, quantifying the percentage of malapposed/uncovered struts, lumen area, stent area, and eventually, the malapposition area and the area of neointimal tissue).[17] Therefore, this allows for better characterization of stent malapposition and lack of coverage.

Automated stent strut segmentation can furthermore be used to achieve a detailed and automatic 3D rendering of stents and vessel wall.[18] This is very important, because 3D intravascular OCT has been shown to be helpful for the optimization of PCI, especially for complex cases such as bifurcation intervention for the rewiring of a jailed branch (Fig. 3). In addition, automatic stent strut segmentation also enables the registration of serial OCT imaging of intracoronary stents over time (Fig. 4),[19] allowing for a very detailed assessment of vessel remodeling over time. Such analyses have been shown to be helpful to better elucidate the mechanisms implicated in the vessel healing procedure following stent implantation.

These methods were typically validated against the gold standard available, which is, in most cases, the manual analysis of stent apposition. In some cases, histopathology (e.g., stent neointimal coverage) has been used as the gold standard.[16] However, in all cases, custom datasets created ad hoc by algorithm developers have been used. To date, there is no common database available for the validation of the different methods for automated stent

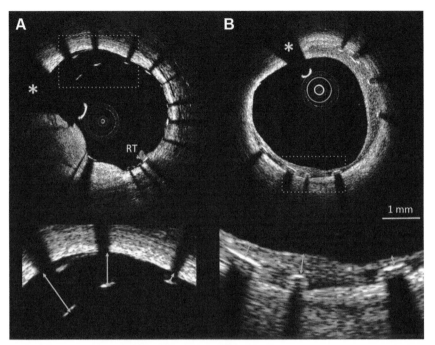

Fig. 2. Quantification on stent strut apposition and coverage. (*A*) How stent strut apposition (malapposition) is typically quantified: the distance between the luminal surface of the strut to the vessel wall is quantified (*yellow arrows*). Similarly, (*B*) shows how stent strut coverage is quantified (*blue arrows*). The asterisk (*) indicates the guidewire shadowing artifact. RT, small residual thrombus on the surface of a strut.

detection. Efforts from the intravascular OCT community are required to achieve a standard procedure for validation, which will be of help to better define the standard requirements. Moreover, this would also enable a detailed comparison of the performances of the different methods proposed in literature, helping the development and selection of optimal approaches for this task. Nevertheless, current methods have been successfully used for the analysis of OCT data, especially to facilitate and speed up core-laboratory activities.[10,20]

Automated Techniques for Plaque Characterization and Segmentation

In addition to stent analysis, one of the main applications of intracoronary OCT imaging is the visualization and assessment of coronary atherosclerotic plaques. OCT has been broadly shown to accurately discriminate the main components of plaques (fibrotic, calcified, and lipid) (Fig. 5).[5,21] However, similarly to stent analysis, the manual assessment of plaques is very inefficient because it is a time-consuming and labor-intensive procedure. Moreover, plaque manual analysis is also subject to interoperator and intraoperator variability. Atherosclerosis is a progressive disease; not in every case can

atherosclerotic tissue be classified into the main plaque components because other types of tissue may be present, such as mixed tissue type, macrophages, cholesterol crystals, and intracoronary thrombus, hampering appropriate analysis.[1]

As such, algorithms for the quantitative characterization of atherosclerotic tissue have been proposed. Because lipid shows a high attenuation coefficient in OCT images, lipid plaques can be detected by attenuation analysis, and algorithms for the automatic quantification of the attenuation coefficient have been proposed,[22] allowing to automatically display areas of high attenuation (e.g., lipid and macrophages) and thus to automatically detect these areas of interest. Following this first approach, other methods have been recently developed to better discriminate between the different plaque types (i.e., fibrotic, calcified, and lipid) by means of image statistical analysis (e.g., texture analysis) combined with tissue attenuation and supervised classification[23] (e.g., Support Vector Machine and Random Forest), statistical models (e.g., Markov model and Bayes Classifier), or other classification algorithms. Moreover, other methods for the fully automated segmentation of calcified plaques based on edge detection have also been proposed.[24]

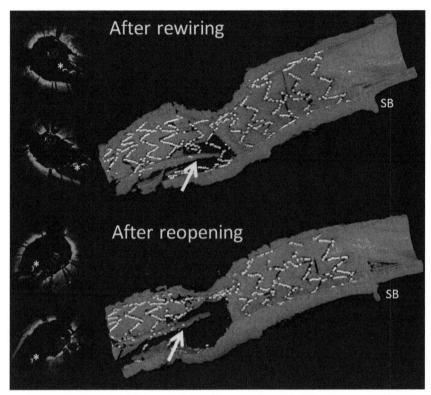

Fig. 3. Fully automated 3D rendering of an intracoronary stent based on the automatic segmentation of stent struts. This kind of 3D view can help to assess which cell of the stent the jailed branch is rewired through (upper 2D image) and the results of the rewiring procedure (lower 3D image), showing optimal results with no free-floating struts over the branch. The *yellow arrows* indicate the position of the guide wire entering the side branch. This kind of analysis may be difficult to obtain by looking at 2D cross-sectional images only. Stent strut segmentation helps for better-quality and more efficient 3D visualization of a stent. The asterisk (*) indicates the guidewire shadowing artifact. SB, side branch. (*From* Ughi GJ, Adriaenssens T, Desmet W, et al. Fully automatic three-dimensional visualization of intravascular optical coherence tomography images: methods and feasibility in vivo. Biomed Opt Express 2012;3:3301; with permission.)

Intravascular OCT analysis of atherosclerotic plaques has several clinical applications. It is an important tool for cardiovascular research (e.g., assessing the effect of drugs and therapies of coronary artery disease) as well as for guiding PCI procedures (e.g., to avoid the placement of stent edges over a thin-cap fibroatheroma).[8] An example of automated plaque analysis of an entire intracoronary OCT pullback is shown in Fig. 6.

In addition to atherosclerotic plaque analysis, it was recently demonstrated that OCT can be used for the characterization of stent neointimal tissue, which is a very important parameter especially for the OCT analysis of drug-eluting stents, because the lack of coverage by mature neointimal tissue has been shown to be a predictor of stent failure.[25] Neointimal tissue covering stent struts can be classified as mature (i.e., including smooth muscle and endothelial cells with interspersed extracellular matrix) versus immature

(i.e., lack of smooth muscle cell and presence of fibrin) based on OCT tissue analysis: immature tissue shows lower backscattering coefficient and more heterogeneity compared with mature tissue. Methods for the automated analysis of stent neointimal tissue, based on statistical image analysis and supervised classification, have been proposed (Fig. 7).[26,27] Such methods in combination with automatic stent strut detection allow for an efficient characterization of stent coverage in vivo.[27]

In most reports, these methods have been validated by comparing them to manual plaque analysis and, in a few cases, by comparison to histopathology. Both approaches show limitations because manual analysis is subject to intraobserver and interobserver variability, and intravascular OCT coregistration to histology is a challenging procedure. Automated tissue characterization and segmentation by intravascular OCT is still in an early stage, and further

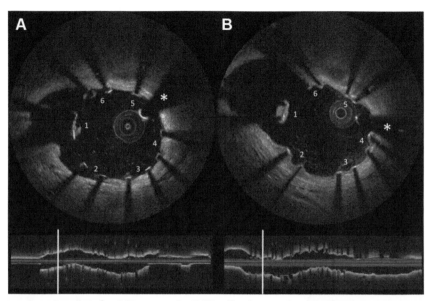

Fig. 4. Automatic registration of serial intravascular OCT pullbacks over time based on automatic stent strut detection (ie, landmark-based registration). (A) Image obtained immediately after drug-eluting stent implantation. (B) Registered image at 9-month follow-up. Numbers 1 to 6 indicate the corresponding regions of interest between the 2 images. (1) Nonapposed struts overlying a side branch; (2) to (5) stent struts registered over time. The asterisk (*) indicates the guidewire shadowing artifact. (Adapted from Ughi GJ, Adriaenssens T, Larsson M, et al. Automatic three-dimensional registration of intravascular optical coherence tomography images. J Biomed Opt 2012;17:026005.)

efforts in the development and standardization from the OCT community to define the requirements for and optimal ways of validation are required. Moreover, additional advancements in intracoronary OCT technology to allow for better discrimination and characterization of atherosclerotic plaques (e.g., multimodality OCT in combination with fluorescence molecular

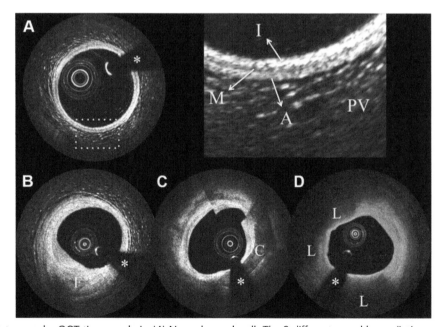

Fig. 5. Intravascular OCT tissue analysis. (A) Normal vessel wall. The 3 different vessel layers (intima, media, and adventitia) surrounded by perivascular tissue are visible. (B) Fibrotic plaque between 6 and 9 o'clock. (C) Calcified plaque between 2 and 6 o'clock. (D) Circumferential lipid plaque (5–12 o'clock). The asterisk (*) indicates the guidewire shadowing artifact. A, adventitia; C, calcified; F, fibrotic; I, intima; L, lipid; M, media; PV, perivascular tissue.

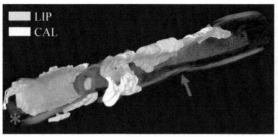
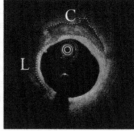

Fig. 6. Automated plaque analysis of an entire intravascular OCT dataset. The *asterisk* indicates the guide wire. The *red arrow* points to a vessel stenosis presenting the IVOCT minimal lumen area. C, calcium; CAL, calcium; L, lipid; LIP, lipid. (*Adapted from* Ughi GJ, Adriaenssens T, Sinnaeve P, et al. Automated tissue characterization of in vivo atherosclerotic plaques by intravascular optical coherence tomography images. Biomed Opt Express 2013;4:1014–30.)

imaging[28] and spectroscopy[29]) may also help in the development of algorithms with higher sensitivity and specificity. Moreover, such advancements could help overcome limitations of current OCT technology, such as the detection and discrimination of necrotic cores, because current OCT and IVUS technology cannot differentiate between lipid and necrotic plaque and enable the reliable assessment of plaque

inflammation, which represents a significant unmet clinical need.

Other Advanced Methods for Intravascular Optical Coherence Tomography Image Analysis

In addition to stent and plaque analysis, other advanced techniques for automated intravascular OCT image processing have been

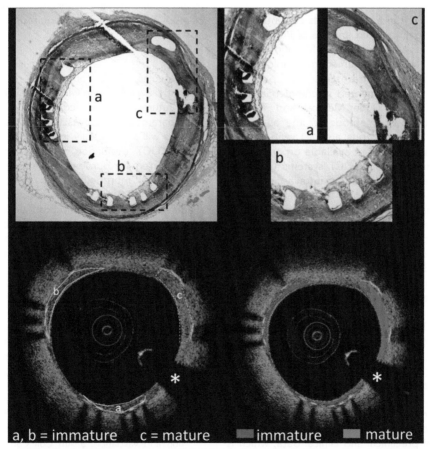

Fig. 7. An example of automated assessment of neointimal tissue maturity. Intravascular OCT images are registered to histopathology and the algorithm validation was obtained accordingly. The asterisk (*) indicates the guidewire shadowing artifact. (*Adapted from* Ughi GJ, Steigerwald K, Adriaenssens T, et al. Automatic characterization of neointimal tissue by intravascular optical coherence tomography. J Biomed Optics 2014;19:21104.)

proposed. Examples include methods for the automated assessment of plaque erosion and intravascular thrombus, and the quantification of macrophage content overlying atherosclerotic plaques.[30–33] Semiautomated methods for the quantification of fibrous cap thickness overlying lipid/necrotic core plaques have been proposed as well as methods for the automatic detection of side branches.[34,35] These additional methods may be of particular help for core-laboratory analyses, in which intravascular OCT is used in large studies aiming to better understand atherosclerotic disease and the safety and efficacy of novel therapies and interventions for coronary artery diseases. To the best of the authors' knowledge, algorithms for the automated detection and quantification of vessel dissections and other interesting artery wall features (e.g., coronary evaginations related to stent implantation[36] and intrastrut cavities[37]) have not been proposed so far.

DISCUSSION

In this article, the main methods currently available for the automated analysis of intravascular OCT images are summarized. Methods for the automatic analysis of lumen morphology and 3D visualization of intravascular OCT pullbacks are currently implemented in commercial OCT systems (i.e., St. Jude Medical and Terumo Corp.). Moreover, methods for the automatic detection of stent struts and 3D rendering of intracoronary stents are available on one of the commercially available OCT systems (i.e., Terumo). The coregistration of intravascular OCT pullbacks to angiography is also available on commercially available systems (i.e., St Jude Medical) and third-party companies have developed specific software for the automated analysis of stent strut apposition/neointimal coverage (e.g., Medis, Leiden, The Netherlands). Similarly, core laboratories and different research groups have developed their own approaches, as illustrated above. However, methods for intravascular OCT tissue characterization and plaque segmentation are not currently commercially available.

Looking forward, there is an unmet need for standardization of the requirements for, and validation of, the various proposed methods. This standardization of the requirements would aid the use of computer-based methods for the analysis of preclinical and clinical data, which is of importance for on-line OCT data analysis as well as for creating a standard for the analysis of such data for core-laboratory activities. This would also allow for a more complete comparison of methods and results between different research groups.

In the near future, the goal of intravascular OCT automated analysis is to provide a comprehensive software package for the automated analysis of lumen morphology, stent strut detection, 3D rendering of vessel wall and implanted devices, and the automatic quantification of stent strut apposition and coverage. This will satisfy the basic needs of the intravascular OCT user, substantially speed up and enhance image analysis for the typical use of OCT technology, and continue to expand the clinical utility of this imaging modality and its use in cardiovascular research.

More advanced image analysis techniques, such as the spatial registration of intravascular OCT datasets and automated plaque characterization and segmentation, may also be widely available in the future. However, automatic tissue analysis is still in its early stage, and to achieve the level of maturity that is needed for routine use, further advancements in intravascular OCT technology are required.

SUMMARY

Intravascular OCT automated analysis is currently available, or will be available in the near future, for the acquisition of standard OCT parameters. Intravascular OCT automated analysis will substantially increase the speed of on-line OCT evaluation for assessments that currently require burdensome manual analyses (e.g., vessel morphology and stent analysis). For computer-aided analysis of atherosclerotic plaques, further technological developments will be required and may be available to the larger OCT community at a later stage. Automatic image analysis is a key requirement to broaden the use of intravascular OCT technology as a clinical tool.

REFERENCES

1. Tearney GJ, Regar E, Akasaka T, et al, International Working Group for Intravascular Optical Coherence Tomography. Consensus standards for acquisition, measurement, and reporting of intravascular optical coherence tomography studies: a report from the international working group for intravascular optical coherence tomography standardization and validation. J Am Coll Cardiol 2012;59: 1058–72.

2. Tearney GJ, Waxman S, Shishkov M, et al. Three-dimensional coronary artery microscopy by

intracoronary optical frequency domain imaging. JACC Cardiovasc Imaging 2008;1:752–61.

3. Bezerra HG, Costa MA, Guagliumi G, et al. Intra-coronary optical coherence tomography: a comprehensive review clinical and research appli-cations. JACC Cardiovasc Interv 2009;2:1035–46.

4. Guagliumi G, Musumeci G, Sirbu V, et al. Optical coherence tomography assessment of in vivo vascular response after implantation of overlapping bare-metal and drug-eluting stents. JACC Cardio-vasc Interv 2010;3:531–9.

5. Yabushita H, Bouma BE, Houser SL, et al. Charac-terization of human atherosclerosis by optical coherence tomography. Circulation 2002;106: 1640–5.

6. Radu M, Jorgensen E, Kelbaek H, et al. Optical coherence tomography at follow-up after percuta-neous coronary intervention: relationship between procedural dissections, stent strut malapposition and stent healing. EuroIntervention 2011;7:353–61.

7. Finn AV, Joner M, Nakazawa G, et al. Pathological correlates of late drug-eluting stent thrombosis: strut coverage as a marker of endothelialization. Circulation 2007;115:2435–41.

8. Waxman S, Freilich MI, Suter MJ, et al. A case of lipid core plaque progression and rupture at the edge of a coronary stent: elucidating the mecha-nisms of drug-eluting stent failure. Circ Cardiovasc Interv 2010;3:193–6.

9. Tanabe K, Serruys PW, Degertekin M, et al. Incom-plete stent apposition after implantation of paclitaxel-eluting stents or bare metal stents: in-sights from the randomized taxus ii trial. Circulation 2005;111:900–5.

10. Adriaenssens T, Dens J, Ughi G, et al. Optical coherence tomography study of healing character-istics of paclitaxel-eluting balloons vs. everolimus-eluting stents for in-stent restenosis: the SEDUCE (Safety and Efficacy of a Drug elUting balloon in Coronary artery rEstenosis) randomised clinical trial. EuroIntervention 2014;10:439–48.

11. Ughi GJ, Adriaenssens T, Onsea K, et al. Automatic segmentation of in-vivo intra-coronary optical coherence tomography images to assess stent strut apposition and coverage. Int J Cardiovasc Imaging 2012;28:229–41.

12. Tsantis S, Kagadis GC, Katsanos K, et al. Automatic vessel lumen segmentation and stent strut detec-tion in intravascular optical coherence tomography. Med Phys 2012;39:503–13.

13. Schmitt JB, Petroff C, Gophinat A, et al. Method and apparatus for automated determination of a lumen contour of a blood vessel. Software. WO/2014/092755. 2013.

14. Lu H, Gargesha M, Wang Z, et al. Automatic stent detection in intravascular oct images using bagged decision trees. Biomed Opt Express 2012;3:2809–24.

15. Kauffmann C, Motreff P, Sarry L. In vivo supervised analysis of stent reendothelialization from optical coherence tomography. IEEE Trans Med Imaging 2010;29:807–18.

16. Ughi GJ, Van Dyck CJ, Adriaenssens T, et al. Auto-matic assessment of stent neointimal coverage by intravascular optical coherence tomography. Eur Heart J Cardiovasc Imaging 2014;15:195–200.

17. Adriaenssens T, Ughi GJ, Dubois C, et al. Auto-mated detection and quantification of clusters of malapposed and uncovered intracoronary stent struts assessed with optical coherence tomogra-phy. Int J Cardiovasc Imaging 2014;30:839–48.

18. Ughi GJ, Dubois C, Desmet W, et al. Provisional side branch stenting: presentation of an automated method allowing online 3D OCT guidance. Eur Heart J Cardiovasc Imaging 2013;14:715.

19. Ughi GJ, Adriaenssens T, Larsson M, et al. Auto-matic three-dimensional registration of intravas-cular optical coherence tomography images. J Biomed Opt 2012;17:026005.

20. De Cock D, Bennett J, Ughi GJ, et al. Healing course of acute vessel wall injury after drug-eluting stent implantation assessed by optical coherence tomography. Eur Heart J Cardiovasc Im-aging 2014;15:800–9.

21. Xu C, Schmitt JM, Carlier SG, et al. Characteriza-tion of atherosclerosis plaques by measuring both backscattering and attenuation coefficients in optical coherence tomography. J Biomed Opt 2008;13:034003.

22. van Soest G, Goderie T, Regar E, et al. Atheroscle-rotic tissue characterization in vivo by optical coher-ence tomography attenuation imaging. J Biomed Opt 2010;15:011105.

23. Ughi GJ, Adriaenssens T, Sinnaeve P, et al. Auto-mated tissue characterization of in vivo atheroscle-rotic plaques by intravascular optical coherence tomography images. Biomed Opt Express 2013;4: 1014–30.

24. Wang Z, Kyono H, Bezerra HG, et al. Semiauto-matic segmentation and quantification of calcified plaques in intracoronary optical coherence tomog-raphy images. J Biomed Opt 2010;15:061711.

25. Malle C, Tada T, Steigerwald K, et al. Tissue charac-terization after drug-eluting stent implantation us-ing optical coherence tomography. Arterioscler Thromb Vasc Biol 2013;33:1376–83.

26. Ughi GJ, Steigerwald K, Adriaenssens T, et al. Automatic characterization of neointimal tissue by intravascular optical coherence tomography. J Biomed Opt 2014;19:21104.

27. Ughi GJ, Adriaenssens T. Automated assessment and 3-dimensional visualization of the pattern of neointimal tissue maturity in vivo following drug-eluting stent implantation. Int J Cardiovasc Imag-ing 2014;30(7):1235–6.

28. Yoo H, Kim JW, Shishkov M, et al. Intra-arterial catheter for simultaneous microstructural and molecular imaging in vivo. Nat Med 2011;17:1680–4.

29. Fard AM, Vacas-Jacques P, Hamidi E, et al. Optical coherence tomography–near infrared spectroscopy system and catheter for intravascular imaging. Opt Express 2013;21:30849–58.

30. Tearney GJ, Yabushita H, Houser SL, et al. Quantification of macrophage content in atherosclerotic plaques by optical coherence tomography. Circulation 2003;107:113–9.

31. Tanaka A, Tearney GJ, Bouma BE. Challenges on the frontier of intracoronary imaging: atherosclerotic plaque macrophage measurement by optical coherence tomography. J Biomed Opt 2010; 15:011104.

32. Tahara S, Morooka T, Wang Z, et al. Intravascular optical coherence tomography detection of atherosclerosis and inflammation in murine aorta. Arterioscler Thromb Vasc Biol 2012;32:1150–7.

33. Wang Z, Jia H, Tian J, et al. Computer-aided image analysis algorithm to enhance in vivo diagnosis of plaque erosion by intravascular optical coherence tomography. Circ Cardiovasc Imaging 2014;7(5): 805–10.

34. Wang Z, Chamie D, Bezerra HG, et al. Volumetric quantification of fibrous caps using intravascular optical coherence tomography. Biomed Opt Express 2012;3:1413–26.

35. Wang A, Eggermont J, Dekker N, et al. 3D assessment of stent cell size and side branch access in intravascular optical coherence tomographic pullback runs. Comput Med Imaging Graph 2014;38: 113–22.

36. Radu MD, Raber L, Kalesan B, et al. Coronary evaginations are associated with positive vessel remodelling and are nearly absent following implantation of newer-generation drug-eluting stents: an optical coherence tomography and intravascular ultrasound study. Eur Heart J 2014;35:795–807.

37. Jama A, Prasad A. Multiple interstrut cavities: a potential mechanism for very late stent thrombosis? Insights from optical coherence tomography. JACC Cardiovasc Interv 2012;5:995–6.

Intravascular Ultrasound for the Diagnosis and Treatment of Left Main Coronary Artery Disease

Jose M. De la Torre Hernandez, MD, PhD, FESC*,
Tamara Garcia Camarero, MD

KEYWORDS

- Left main coronary artery • Coronary artery disease • Angiography • Intravascular ultrasound
- Percutaneous coronary intervention • Drug-eluting stents

KEY POINTS

- Intravascular ultrasound (IVUS) is helpful in the assessment of left main coronary artery (LMCA) lesion severity, overcoming the multiple limitations of angiography within this anatomic segment.
- IVUS provides information about atherosclerotic burden, plaque extension, and plaque morphology from the aorto–ostial junction to the distal segment, and the ostia of the left anterior descending and left circumflex arteries.
- With other clinical data, a minimum lumen area cutoff of 6 mm^2 can inform and provide guidance with regard to deferral of revascularization.
- IVUS can be help to plan percutaneous interventions (PCI) and optimize the results with respect to stent size, lesion coverage, stent apposition, expansion, and the detection of edge dissection.
- IVUS guidance of LMCA PCI with drug-eluting stents has been shown to improve clinical outcomes, particularly in patients with distal left main disease.

LIMITATIONS OF ANGIOGRAPHY FOR LEFT MAIN ASSESSMENT

The left main coronary artery (LMCA) is critical segment in the coronary tree, because it supplies a large majority of the left ventricular myocardium; in the setting of left dominance, the left main contributes nearly its entire blood supply. Therefore, an accurate assessment of coronary disease at this site, as well as the most optimized percutaneous coronary intervention (PCI) result, is crucial for clinical outcomes. Standard contrast angiography has been and remains essential in the assessment of the coronary tree, including the LMCA. However, although angiography is highly accurate when defining critical or very severely obstructive lesions, its precision declines when contrast filling defects or intermediate stenosis are involved. Furthermore, noncoaxial alignment and a deficient or excessive catheter engagement result in a loss of diagnostic power.

J.M. de la Torre Hernandez has received grants for research from Abbott Vascular, Boston Scientific, Biosensors, St Jude, and Biotronik. He has received payments for advisory and presentations from Abbott Vascular, Boston Scientific, Biosensors, St Jude, Biotronik, Volcano, Lilly and AstraZeneca.
Interventional Cardiology Department, Unidad de Cardiología Intervencionista, Hospital Universitario Marques de Valdecilla, Valdecilla Sur, Santander 39008, Spain
* Corresponding author. Unidad de Hemodinámica y Cardiología Intervencionista, Hospital Universitario Marqués de Valdecilla, Valdecilla Sur, Santander 39008, Spain.
E-mail address: he1thj@humv.es

Other contributors to diagnostic inaccuracy include the diffuse nature of the coronary artery disease, expansive or constrictive remodeling, ostial or bifurcational involvement, calcification, eccentric plaque formation, and superimposition or overlap of branches. The limitations of angiography are illustrated by the high degree of interobserver variability in angiographic interpretation of coronary lesions.[1,2]

The interpretation of LMCA obstruction by angiography is particularly fraught with these problems, compounded by its short segment, the fact that the aorto–ostial junction is usually nonperpendicular to the lumen axis, and the frequent involvement of plaque within the distal bifurcation or trifurcation. Owing to its short span, LMCA disease usually involves the entire length of the vessel, and there is no "nondiseased" referent segment. This can result in an underestimation of the disease burden by angiography. Vessel remodeling can affect the entire left main or only a portion of it. Therefore, angiography can overestimate the amount of plaque in the case of constrictive remodeling (more frequent in the ostium) or underestimate it in the case of expansive remodeling. The catheter position over the ostium and the contrast jet can create angiographic artifacts that usually result in the appearance of a falsely severe ostial stenosis. The catheter may bend the left main (especially if it is not diseased), making it seem to be stenotic (Fig. 1). Coronary sinus opacification can interfere with LMCA visualization. The angle of the left main bifurcation has substantial variability, and sometimes branches are overlapped and impede angiographic assessment of the severity of distal obstruction. Calcification can create nodular contrast defects that impede proper lumen assessment. Moreover, underneath these lumen defects can reside not only calcified nodules, but also ruptured plaques or thrombi. All of these issues with left main angiography result in interobserver angiographic variability, poor correlation with postmortem histology, and poor correlation with in vivo intravascular ultrasound (IVUS) studies. Indeed, in the Coronary Artery Study (CASS) study, the LMCA segment had the greatest interobserver variability of the coronary tree, and substantial variability in stenosis severity was observed between the core laboratory and local site investigators.[2] When comparing angiography post-mortem histopathology, angiography underestimated one-half of the lesions that were histologically severe and overestimated one-half of the lesions that were histologically mild.[3,4]

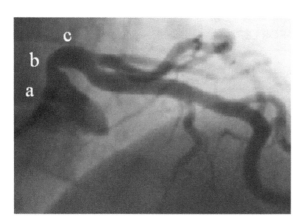
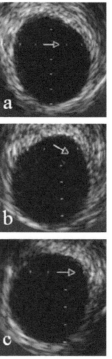

Fig. 1. Angiographic artifact. False stenosis at the left main midshaft (bending by the catheter). Sites demarcated with a, b, c on angiographic image correlate with intravascular ultrasound images (a), (b), and (c). *Arrow*, axis for longitudinal imaging reconstruction.

IVUS studies also confirm this lack of correlation between angiographic severity and actual lumen area: in the LITRO (estudio de Lesiones Intermedias de TROnco) study, wide scatter was observed in angiographic parameters between groups with left main minimal luminal area less than or at least 6 mm², which has been validated as an optimal IVUS-based cutoff for significant lesion severity (Fig. 2).

THE ROLE OF INTRAVASCULAR ULTRASOUND FOR THE ASSESSMENT OF LEFT MAIN CORONARY ARTERY LESION SEVERITY

IVUS was first used in the assessment of LMCA lesions in the 1990s, and illustrative cases were reported suggesting that IVUS was able to detect a greater degree of disease compared with angiography.[5–7] Nevertheless, the first and landmark study was reported by the Washington Heart Center,[8] in which a total of 122 patients without severe left main lesions by angiography were assessed with IVUS. At 1-year follow-up, the IVUS-derived minimum lumen diameter was the strongest independent predictor of clinical events, in addition to diabetes and the presence of nontreated lesions in other vessels. A subsequent study supported these findings.[9]

However, these studies did not use a prespecified IVUS cutoff value to decide whether the LMCA lesion was severe, and most of the clinical events in the follow-up were revascularizations decided by the clinician. Subsequently, other studies have sought to define an IVUS criterion to be chosen as cutoff value of an ischemia-generating left main lesion (Table 1). Different strategies to ascertain such a cutoff include correlating IVUS-derived parameters with fractional flow reserve (FFR), defining a "normal" IVUS value based on a patient population with no or mild left main disease, and calculating a theoretic normal minimal luminal area from fractal mathematics applied to the coronary tree.

Correlation of Intravascular Ultrasound Parameters with Fractional Flow Reserve

Several studies have evaluated the correlation between IVUS findings and FFR measurements across LMCA lesions. In 1 study, 55 patients with intermediate LMCA lesions were assessed both with FFR and IVUS.[10] According to receiver operator characteristic curve analysis, a minimal luminal diameter of less than 2.8 mm had the highest sensitivity, specificity, and accuracy (93%, 98%, and 96%, respectively) to predict an FFR of less than 0.75, followed by a minimum

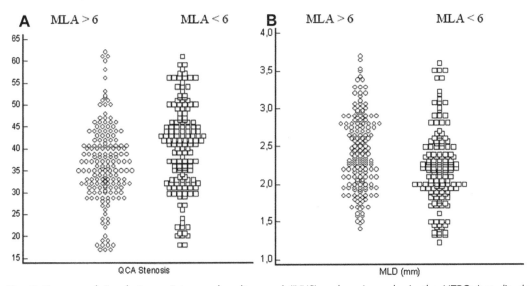

Fig. 2. Poor correlation between intravascular ultrasound (IVUS) and angiography in the LITRO (estudio de Lesiones Intermedias de TROnco) study. (A) Box and whisker comparison graph for angiographic left main coronary artery stenosis in both IVUS-derived groups. (B) Box and whisker comparison graph for angiographic left main coronary artery minimum lumen diameter in both IVUS-derived groups. MLA, minimal lumen area; MLD, minimal lumen diameter; QCA, quantitative coronary angiography. Circles, deferred group; squares, revascularized group. (From De la Torre Hernandez JM, Hernandez Hernandez F, Alfonso F, et al. Prospective application of Pre-defined intravascular ultrasound criteria for assessment of intermediate left main coronary artery lesions results from the multicenter LITRO study. J Am Coll Cardiol 2011;58:354; with permission.)

Table 1
Proposed published cutoff values for LMCA
MLA

Table 1
Proposed published cutoff values for LMCA MLA

Study	Methods	Cutoff MLA (mm²)
Park et al,[11] 2014	IVUS vs FFR <0.8; n = 112	4.5
Jasti et al,[10] 2004	IVUS vs FFR <0.75; n = 55	5.9
Fassa et al,[13] 2005	Population based normal range; n = 214	7.5
De la Torre Hernandez et al,[16] 2011	Prospective clinical validation; n = 354	6

Abbreviations: FFR, fractional flow reserve; MLA, minimal lumen area.

lumen area (MLA) of less than 5.9 mm², which had a sensitivity, specificity, and accuracy of 93%, 95%, and 94%, respectively. Patients were revascularized according to the FFR findings, and the survival at 38 months of follow-up was 100% in both the deferred (n = 37) and the treated (n = 14) groups; major event-free survival was 90% and 100%, respectively.[10] In a more recent study of 112 patients with indeterminate LMCA disease, the optimal IVUS cutoff to predict an FFR of 0.80 or less was an MLA of less than 4.5 mm², which provided 77% sensitivity, 82% specificity, 84% positive predictive value, and a 75% negative predictive value.[11] A metaanalysis including studies that assessed the correlation of IVUS and FFR in a variety of coronary lesions found that the predictive power of an absolute MLA cutoff by IVUS differed across LMCA and non-LMCA lesions. MLA had limited accuracy in non-LMCA lesions, whereas for intermediate LMCA lesions, the IVUS-derived MLA had a 90% sensitivity and 90% specificity to predict an FFR of less than 0.8.[12] The greater agreement between IVUS-derived MLA and FFR for LMCA lesions compared with non-LMCA lesions may be owing to the limited variability in LMCA length, the greater size of the LMCA, and the limited variability in the amount of myocardium that the LMCA supplies.

Left Main Luminal Area in Patient Population with No Stenosis

The Mayo Clinic study aimed to determine the reference left main MLA of their population.[13] To do so, they assessed by IVUS the MLA of 121 consecutive patients with angiographically normal LMCA and defined the lower range of the LMCA MLA as the mean -2 standard deviations (SD), which resulted in a value of 7.5 mm². In another phase of the study, they assessed 214 consecutive patients with intermediate LMCA lesions by IVUS. A total of 131 patients were found to have an MLA of greater than 7.5 mm², and in 114 (89%) revascularization was deferred. The remaining 83 patients had an MLA of less than 7.5 mm² and 71 (85.5%) were treated. After a mean follow-up of 3 years, there were no differences in the cardiac adverse event rate between the groups. There are several limitations of this study; an angiographically normal LMCA does not exclude the presence of disease, the cutoff value might have been influenced by the population profile, the use of the mean -2 SD as the lower range of normal is controversial. Finally, and there was incomplete adherence to the protocol (<90%).

Predicted Left Main Luminal Area Estimated Using Fractal Mathematics

The coronary vasculature follows fractal principles, and therefore is possible to calculate the theoretic size of a parent vessel knowing the size of its daughter branches. In the particular case of the LMCA, Finet and colleagues[14] concluded that the most accurate approach to perform this calculation would be the Linear law, in which diameter [parent vessel] = 0.678 (diameter [daughter 1] + diameter [daughter 2]), rather than the Murray's law, which would underestimate the parent vessel size, or the flow preservation law, which would overestimate it. Assuming a threshold value of 3 mm² for the proximal segment of both left main branches (based on FFR and IVUS correlation studies), the predicted MLA of the LMCA is approximately 5.8 mm². Of note, a more recent study has found that the HK model would provide valid calculations for every bifurcation.[15]

Prospective, Clinical Validation of the Intravascular Ultrasound–Derived Minimum Lumen Area Cutoff Value for Left Main Lesion

Although a mathematically predicted MLA cutoff value of the LMCA or values derived from correlations between IVUS and FFR are helpful, it is critical to demonstrate that a proposed cutoff is safe clinically. This was the rationale of the design the LITRO (estudio de Lesiones Intermedias de TROnco) study.[16] A pilot study initially assessed the safety of applying an IVUS LMCA MLA cutoff of 6.0 mm² or less in 79 patients. In 48 patients, the LMCA MLA was greater than 6 mm², so the LMCA was left untreated. At a mean follow-up of 40 months, only two of these patients required revascularization.[17] At a mean of 8 years follow-up, only 2 of the 48 patients (4.2%) in the deferral group (MLA >6 mm^2) have required revascularization.[18] In the larger LITRO study, a total of 22 Spanish hospitals prospectively enrolled 354 patients with intermediate LMCA lesions assessed with IVUS. Lesions with MLA of less than 6 mm^2 were recommended to be treated, whereas deferral was recommended for those lesions with MLA of 6 mm^2 or greater.[16] The LMCA MLA was 6 mm^2 or greater in 186 patients and among them 179 (96%) were left untreated (deferred group). The LMCA MLA was less than 6 mm^2 in the remaining 168 patients, and 152 (90%) of them treated with either PCI or coronary artery bypass grafting (revascularized group). Angiography discriminated between these 2 groups poorly (see **Fig. 2**): the MLA was less than 6 mm^2 in 33% of patients with angiographic stenosis less than 30%, whereas the MLA was 6 mm^2 or greater in 43% of patients with angiographic stenosis greater than 50%. At the 2-year follow-up, clinical outcomes were similar in both the deferred and revascularized groups. Survival free from cardiac death was 97.7% in the deferred group compared with 94.5% in the revascularized group ($P = .5$) and survival free from cardiac death, infarction, and any revascularization was 87.3% versus 80.6%, respectively ($P = .3$; **Fig. 3**). The need for left main revascularization in the deferred group was low (4.4%) and none of the patients presented with a myocardial infarction. Of note, the 16 patients with an LMCA MLA between 5 and 6 mm^2 whom did not undergo revascularization had worse clinical outcomes: the rate of major adverse cardiovascular events rate for this group was 31.2% compared with 5.6% for the 53 patients with MLAs between 6 and 7.5 mm^2.

Rationale for a proposed minimum lumen area cutoff of 6 mm^2

Although the published data are somewhat disparate regarding a proposed MLA cutoff for a significant LMCA lesion, we propose that an MLA of greater than 6 mm^2 is a safe and appropriate cutoff for which to defer LMCA revascularization based upon the following considerations.

First, the LMCA MLA cutoff seems to be population dependent. A study within the United States yielded an optimal cutoff value of 5.9 mm^2 (sensitivity, 93%; specificity, 94%) for an FFR of less than 0.75,[10] whereas a study conducted in South Korea provided a lower value of 4.5 mm^2.[11] The average MLA of the LMCAs in

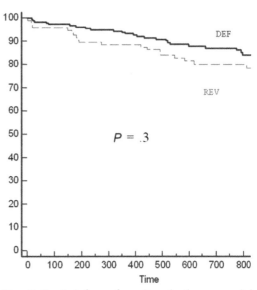

Fig. 3. Survival free of cardiac death, myocardial infarction and any revascularization in groups with left main coronary artery revascularized and deferred revascularization in the LITRO study. DEF, deferral group; REV, revascularized group. (*From* De la Torre Hernandez JM, Hernandez Hernandez F, Alfonso F, et al. Prospective application of Pre-defined intravascular ultrasound criteria for assessment of intermediate left main coronary artery lesions results from the multicenter LITRO study. J Am Coll Cardiol 2011;58:357; with permission.)

the patients included in these 2 studies are strikingly different: 7.6 mm^2 in the US study compared with 4.8 mm^2 in the Korean study. The most plausible explanation for such differences seems to be related to ethnicity. Another study compared LMCA lesions between 99 Caucasian patients from North America and 99 Asian patients. Asian patients had a significantly smaller LMCA MLA (5.2 ± 1.8 vs 6.2 ± 1.4 mm^2; $P<.0001$).[19] Accordingly, we believe that the attempts by Park and colleagues[11] to adjust for body mass index in their series of 112 Asian-only patients cannot exclude this important influence. Second, given the unique prognostic implications of LMCA-derived ischemia, the optimal cutoff point must provide very high sensitivity and negative predictive value to be clinically acceptable. For an LMCA MLA cutoff of 4.5 mm^2, the sensitivity has been shown to be 77% and the negative predictive value 75%, which are clearly suboptimal for clinical decision making. Notably, among the 54 lesions with an LMCA MLA of greater than 4.5 mm^2, 13 lesions (24.1%) had an FFR of at least 0.80 mm^2. We believe that missing 1 out of 4 patients with severe ischemia is not acceptable for an LMCA lesion. In comparison, a cutoff of 6 mm^2 is more acceptable clinically.[10,11] In the multicenter LITRO study, we found that in patients with an LMCA MLA of at least 6 mm^2, revascularization could be safely deferred.[16] We suggest that an LMCA MLA of between 5 and 6 mm^2 should be considered a diagnostic "gray area" in which clinical decisions should be individualized or, potentially, complemented with FFR evaluation if feasible.

Third, a theoretic LMCA MLA cutoff value can be derived from fractal geometry. A study confirmed that the Linear law was more exact in this regard than Murray's law, which underestimated the calculated mother vessel diameter.[14] Using the currently established 3 mm^2 as the best cutoff MLA for the LMCA branches,[20] the calculated left main–MLA cutoff by the Linear law is 5.8 mm^2, similar to the proposed cutpoint of 6.0 mm^2.

Fourth, the optimal LMCA MLA cutoff value should be validated prospectively. In LITRO,[16] a prospective multicenter study including 354 patients, the 6 mm^2 cutoff value was validated clinically. At 2 years, the outcome of deferred patients was equivalent to that of the revascularized group. Importantly, was significantly worse in the few patients with LMCA MLAs between 5 and 6 mm^2.

Therefore, we believe that a proposed MLA of 4.5 mm^2 as the optimal LMCA MLA cutoff value should be taken cautiously until further clinical data support its prognostic validity. The IVUS-obtained MLA of an LMCA lesion is only 1 data point to incorporate into clinical decision making, along with many other clinical and angiographic variables. The MLA cutpoint of 6 mm^2 should be considered to be more of an exclusion criterion to define when revascularization should not be performed (ie, defer when MLA $\geq$6 mm^2) rather than a value that entails the absolute need for revascularization on its own (Fig. 4). An important observation studies of deferred revascularization in patients with adequate LMCA MLA is that the average baseline MLA of the patients whom incur events after deferred revascularization is not usually just around the borderline of the cutoff (mean MLA in patients with events after deferral, 8.4 $\pm$ 2 mm^2 in De la Torre Hernandez and colleagues,[16] 7.2 $\pm$ 2.2 mm^2 in Okabe and colleagues,[21] and 6.8 $\pm$ 4.4 mm^2 in Abizaid and colleagues[8]). Therefore, many of these events may have no causal relation to the initial LMCA lesion or that progression of disease at the LMCA level and subsequent luminal narrowing may occur abruptly, as in the other coronary locations (Fig. 5).

Intravascular Ultrasound or Fractional Flow Reserve for Left Main Assessment

IVUS and FFR are both safe methods to assess the severity of ambiguous left main lesions, but they have specific advantages and limitations. One potential limitation of IVUS assessment for LMCA severity is the population variability in the average size of the LCMA, which should not affect FFR assessment. However, there are several issues that may affect FFR measurement in the setting of LMCA stenosis, including significant, concomitant left anterior descending artery (LAD) and/or left circumflex significant

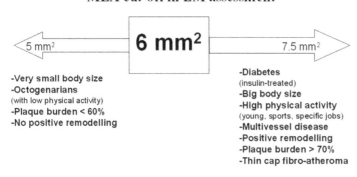

Fig. 4. There is a narrow range for the left main (LM) coronary artery minimal lumen area (MLA) cutoff of about 6 mm^2. Incorporation of other factors is required to make an individualized, case-based decision.

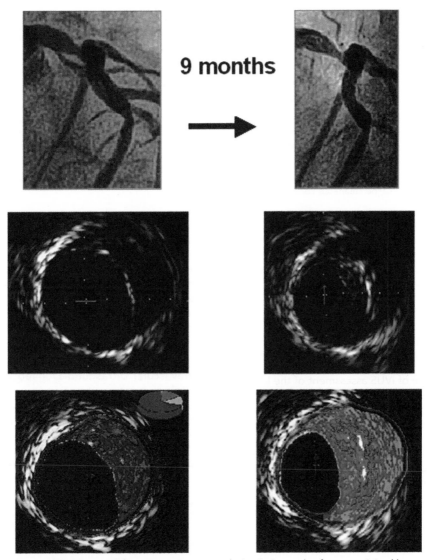

Fig. 5. Progression of disease in a left main coronary artery lesion in 9 months, from an minimal lumen area (MLA) of 10.4 mm^2 and 59% plaque burden to an MLA of 5.7 mm^2 and 75% plaque burden.

disease is frequent (30%–40% of cases)[22]; collaterals to an occluded or subtotally occluded right coronary artery; interindividual variation in hyperemic response to adenosine; vulnerability to technical issues such as drift, equalization, and so on; and uncertainty regarding the gray zone between 0.75 and 0.80. On the other hand, the correlation between FFR and IVUS correlation for LMCA lesions is greater than for non-LMCA lesions, as noted.[12]

An important advantage of IVUS compared with FFR for LMCA evaluation is the ability to obtain key morphologic information, such as characterization of the severity and extent of disease (eg, ostial LAD and/or ostial left circumflex involvement, calcification that may require

atherectomy). Importantly, plaque burden was the only predictor of events at the 5-year follow-up for LMCA lesions left untreated.[21]

The strengths and limitations of IVUS and FFR to assess the severity of ambiguous left main lesions are summarized in Table 2. It may be useful to select the modality of basal LMCA assessment based on several criteria. For example, FFR may be preferred (with secondary use of IVUS) in the presence of isolated ostial or midshaft LMCA lesions in patients who are more appropriate candidates for coronary artery bypass grafting rather than PCI. IVUS may be the preferred modality in the setting of a distal LMCA bifurcation lesion, diffuse distal disease involving the left anterior descending, and/or left circumflex

Table 2
Strengths and limitations of IVUS and FFR for the evaluation of ambiguous left main stenosis

	IVUS	Fractional Flow Reserve
Strengths	Provides additional anatomic information in the case of subsequent PCI	Cutoff value applies across population and vessel sizes
Limitations	Definite, universal cutoff value not available	Lack of anatomic information
	Narrow range of MLA for LMCA around 6 mm^2, and incorporation of other factors required to make a patient-specific decision	Reliability unclear in the presence of severe LAD and/or left circumflex disease

Abbreviations: IVUS, intravascular ultrasound; LAD, left anterior descending; LMCA, left main coronary artery; MLA, minimal luminal area; PCI, percutaneous coronary intervention.

arteries, and likely candidates for PCI. FFR assessment after IVUS may be considered in the setting of an MLA between 5 and 6 mm^2 in select cases such as individuals with very small body size or in the very elderly.

BASELINE CHARACTERIZATION BY INTRAVASCULAR ULTRASOUND OF ATHEROMATOUS DISEASE INVOLVING THE LEFT MAIN CORONARY ARTERY

The purpose of IVUS assessment of the LMCA is to not only define the severity of the lesion, but also to provide morphologic features of the disease process. This assessment can be helpful to guide any subsequent percutaneous revascularization procedure. Certain morphologic features of the lesion, such as severe circumferential calcification, may dissuade the operator from performing a PCI and opting instead for coronary artery bypass grafting, or can help to establish the most appropriate technical approach to PCI.

Basic Intravascular Ultrasound Information to Obtain During Assessment of Left Main
In every left main lesion
Angiographic characterization of LMCA disease is far from perfect, particularly for ostial and distal lesions. Frequently, IVUS demonstrates that ostial stenosis that seems significant by angiography is actually not present. Angiography suffers from several limitations in assessing the individual involvement of left anterior descending or left circumflex ostia, and does not classify properly distal LMCA lesions. Distal LMCA lesions are the most prevalent and also the most complex to characterize and treat. Left main length is associated with the characteristics of plaque distribution: LMCAs less than 10 mm in length have more ostial involvement, whereas longer LMCAs are prone to develop the plaque within the more distal portion.[23] Ostial lesions often present with a greater degree of constrictive remodeling, less

plaque burden, and less calcification.[16] IVUS studies demonstrate that significant atherosclerotic involvement of the carina is rare, and the plaque observed within the distal LMCA usually extends to both branches, although left anterior descending is more often involved (90%) than left circumflex (62%).[24] Box 1 and Table 3 summarize the information that should be collected uniformly during IVUS assessment of the LMCA.

Intravascular Ultrasound–Derived Virtual Histology
IVUS-derived radiofrequency analysis allows some degree of in vivo arterial histopathology characterization. Plaques located in the LMCA generally carry minimal necrotic content. Thus, they mimic the distal but not the proximal segment of the

Box 1
Intravascular ultrasound parameters that should be collected during diagnostic assessment of the ambiguous left main coronary artery lesion

Luminal area along the length of the LMCA (from distal bifurcation to ostium)

MLA

Plaque burden at site of MLA

Calcification at site of MLA

Diffuse of focal distribution of plaque

Additional parameters in the setting of distal LMCA lesion

Ostial-proximal LAD lumen area, plaque area, and calcification

Ostial-proximal LCX lumen area, plaque area, and calcification

Abbreviations: LAD, left anterior descending artery; LCX, left circumflex artery; LMCA, left main coronary artery; MLA, minimal lumen area.

Table 3
Intravascular ultrasound parameters for clinical decision making once PCI is selected as therapeutic modality

Parameter	Influence on PCI Decision Making
Evaluation of site of angiographic haziness or filling defect	Calcium, thrombus, or dissection?
Severity and distribution of calcification	Need for rotational atherectomy
Luminal and vessel areas as well as plaque burden in the selected landing sites	Selection of stent length and diameter
Severity of disease at ostial LCX	Provisional stenting or dedicated 2-stent approach?
Severity of disease, plaque distribution and lumen-vessel size at LAD, LCX, and LMCA	Selection of best-suited 2-stent technique

Abbreviations: LAD, left anterior descending artery; LCX, left circumflex; LMCA, left main coronary artery; PCI, percutaneous coronary intervention.

left coronary artery, where plaque rupture or vessel occlusion occurs more frequently.[25]

Thin cap fibroatheroma was present more frequently in the proximal LAD than LMCA, supporting the notion that plaque rupture occurs in nonuniform locations throughout the coronary tree and preferentially spares the LMCA.[26]

CHARACTERIZATION OF LEFT MAIN IN-STENT RESTENOSIS AND ITS THERAPEUTIC IMPLICATIONS

In addition to the evaluation of de novo disease, IVUS assessment is helpful for the evaluation of LMCA in-stent restenosis. Distal lesions are more prone to restenosis, which usually occurs at the level of the left circumflex ostium. There are several key aspects of IVUS evaluation that help to elucidate the mechanism(s) of restenosis and suggest the best treatment strategy: confirmation that there is appropriate stent coverage at the site of angiographic restenosis (in particular, the ostium of the LMCA or the ostium of the left circumflex after 2-stent technique); identify stent underexpansion, if present; evaluate for neointimal hyperplasia or in-stent neoatherosclerosis; exclude the presence of stent fracture.

INTRAVASCULAR ULTRASOUND FOR PROCEDURAL PLANNING AND OPTIMIZATION OF LEFT MAIN PERCUTANEOUS CORONARY INTERVENTION
Procedural Planning
Need for plaque modification techniques before predilatation
The presence of superficial annular calcification can suggest the need for rotational ablation. In

acute or unstable lesions, a contrast filling defect can correspond to thrombus, plaque disruption or nodular calcium (**Fig. 6**). In the case of thrombus, aspiration may be required to prevent embolization with predilatation.

Nondistal lesions: selection of stent length and diameter
In nondistal lesions, the length of LMCA that needs to be covered and the appropriate stent diameter can be defined by IVUS. The disease usually is diffuse in nature and focal LMCA stenosis can be associated with a substantial degree of plaque burden involving the remainder of the vessel. If the edge of the stent is deployed within these areas, the risk for edge dissection/hematoma and large residual plaque increases, with a subsequent higher probability of stent thrombosis and restenosis. IVUS can be used to help select the most suitable landing sites.

In ostial lesions, constrictive, or negative, remodeling is usually present. IVUS can be used to define the actual vessel diameter and to establish safely the maximum stent diameter to be used. Midshaft LMCA lesions need to have the ostium well evaluated to decide whether the stent needs to cover the aorto–ostial junction, which may not be clear angiographically. Similarly, IVUS can inform whether the stent should be extended into the LAD for severe midshaft LMCA lesions associated with moderate distal disease.

Distal lesions: technique and stent selection
Distal LMCA lesions are the most frequently encountered (70%–80%) and, compared with ostial or midshaft lesions, more complex to assess and treat. To estimate the precise extension of stent coverage, the midshaft and LMCA ostium must be evaluated.

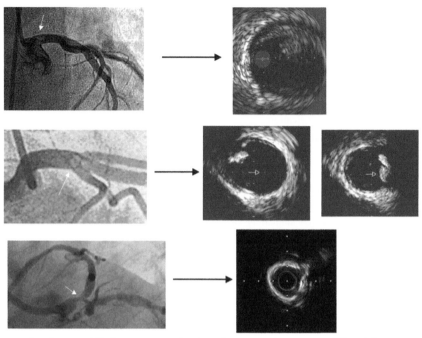

Fig. 6. Intravascular ultrasound findings upon evaluation of angiographic contrast-filling defects.

It is necessary to define separately the involvement of left anterior descending and left circumflex ostia. When there is no significant plaque at the left circumflex ostium, a single stent approach from the LMCA into the left anterior descending might be chosen (Fig. 7). A preprocedural minimal lumen area of less than 3.7 mm² within the left circumflex

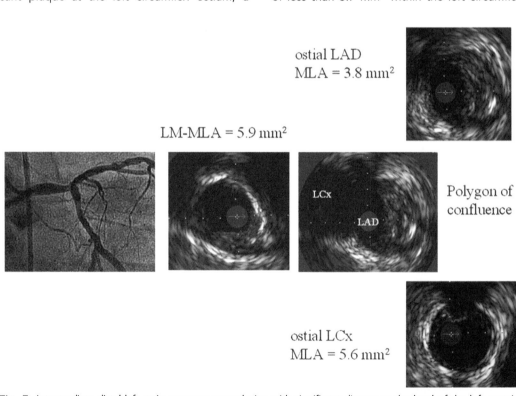

Fig. 7. Intermediate distal left main coronary artery lesion with significant disease at the level of the left anterior descending (LAD) ostium but not within the ostial left circumflex. LCx, left circumflex; LM, left main; MLA, minimal lumen area.

ostium was predictive of a post-stenting FFR of less than 0.80 (sensitivity, 100%; specificity, 71%; positive predictive value, 16%; negative predictive value, 100%). A preprocedural plaque burden of greater than 56% at the left circumflex ostium also predicted a post-stenting FFR of less than 0.80, with a sensitivity of 100%, specificity of 65%, a positive predictive of 14%, and a negative predictive value of 100%.[27] Therefore, a left circumflex ostium with MLA greater than 3.5 to 4 mm^2 and/or plaque burden of less than 50% to 55% can be used as IVUS criteria to select with provisional stenting approach with crossing over of the left circumflex (Fig. 8).

When both the left anterior descending and left circumflex ostia have significant disease, a 2-stent approach might be needed. This approach is recommended in presence of significant or complicated plaques in the LCx ostium (MLA <3.5–4 mm^2 and plaque burden >50%–55%) with extension of disease beyond 5 mm

from the ostium into the proximal left circumflex (Fig. 9). IVUS can help to determine the length and diameter of both stents. IVUS parameters can also help to guide the selection of the particular 2-stent technique to be used. If the LMCA body has a wide lumen and the plaque resides mainly at the bifurcation and/or both ostia, then the V kissing or the minicrush technique is an appropriate choice (Fig. 10). If the LMCA–left anterior descending stent has to cover the midshaft or reach the aorto–ostial junction, then the culotte, minicrush, T, and T-and-protrusion techniques could be useful. When the angle between the left circumflex and the LMCA is close to 90°, the T stenting and T-and-protrusion techniques can be suitable. In cases with a narrower angle, a culotte, mini-crush, and T-and-Protrusion approaches can be appropriate. Critical luminal composed of the left circumflex lumen might suggest the implantation of a stent in the left circumflex followed by the LMCA-left anterior descending stent. Box 2 summarizes

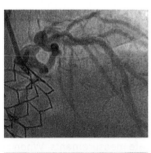
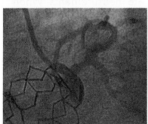
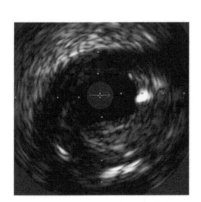

LM-MLA = 4.9 mm^2

ostial LAD
MLA = 5.5 mm^2

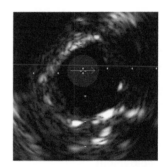

ostial LCx
MLA = 5.8 mm^2

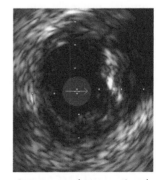

Fig. 8. Intermediate distal left main coronary artery lesion in a patient with previous transcatheter aortic valve replacement. Significant involvement of distal left main but not within the ostial left anterior descending or left circumflex. LAD, left anterior descending; LCx, left circumflex; LM, left main; MLA, minimal lumen area.

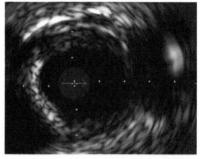

ostial LAD
MLA = 7 mm²

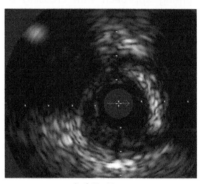

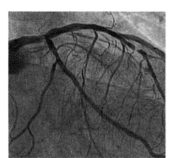

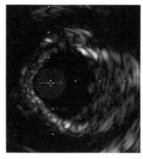

LM-MLA = 4.7 mm²

ostial LCx
MLA = 3.2 mm²

Fig. 9. Intermediate lesion of the distal left main coronary artery (LMCA) with severe lesion in the mid left anterior descending (LAD). Intravascular ultrasound shows significant lumen narrowing of the distal LMCA and also the ostial left circumflex (LCx). LM, left main; MLA, minimal lumen area.

the recommendations for the selection of provisional or 2-stent techniques.

Intravascular Ultrasound Assessment of Left Main Coronary Artery After Stent Deployment

Appropriate lesion coverage and stent edges
For ostial lesions, IVUS can confirm whether the stent covers the entire ostium properly and if it protrudes minimally into the aorta (Fig. 11). For midshaft LMCA lesions, IVUS helps to detect edge problems (ie, dissection, hematoma, large residual plaque). For distal lesions treated with 2 stents, IVUS allows a proper assessment of distal edges (at the level of the left anterior descending and left circumflex) and the proximal edge (at the level of the LMCA).

Stent apposition
This role of IVUS to enhance and confirm stent apposition is relevant particularly in the treatment of distal LMCA lesions. The diameter of the LMCA to left anterior descending artery stent is determined usually by the lumen area

of proximal LAD lumen (which is generally smaller than the proximal reference lumen at the level of the LMCA). This size is underestimated by angiography whereas IVUS can obtain more accurate and safe measurements. When an important difference is present between the reference proximal LMCA lumen and the reference distal left anterior descending artery lumen, some degree of incomplete stent apposition may be observed, which can be detected with IVUS and treated.

Stent expansion
The degree of stent expansion and the minimum intra-stent lumen obtained can be assessed with IVUS. Some ostial lesions, which are often quite very fibrotic, need to be postdilated with noncompliant balloons. Contrast streaming prevents precise angiographic evaluation of stent expansion at the aorto–ostial junction. With distal LMCA lesions, adequate stent expansion is very important, because these portend a higher risk of restenosis and even thrombosis. It is necessary to assess the stent expansion at the

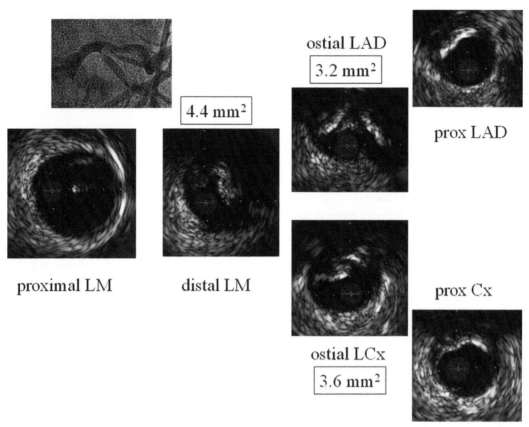

Fig. 10. Calcified lesion within the distal left main coronary artery with haziness and irregular lumen on coronary angiography. Calcification is nodular and amenable to being treated with angioplasty. Both ostia of the left anterior descending (LAD) and left circumflex (LCx) are significantly affected. LM, left main.

level of the LMCA, at the level of the "polygon of confluence" (merger of the left anterior and left circumflex arteries, and at the level of the ostia of the left anterior descending and left circumflex (Fig. 12). The predictive value of the minimum intrastent lumen area at these 4 sites for subsequent clinical events was explored in a study of 403 patients with distal LMCA lesions that underwent IVUS-guided PCI and had 9-month angiographic followup.[28] The optimal MLA cutoff values to predict restenosis were 8 mm^2 at the level of the LMCA, 7 mm^2 at the polygon of confluence, 6 mm^2 at the ostium of the left anterior descending, and 5 mm^2 at the ostium of the left circumflex. Using these criteria, 133 patients (33.8%) had underexpansion of 1 or more segments. Underexpansion was more frequent in the group of patients receiving 2 stents compared with a single stent (54% vs 27%, respectively; P = .001). In the 2-stent group, the left circumflex ostium was the most common site of underexpansion (37%), which may explain the greater risk of restenosis when

LMCA bifurcation lesions are treated with a 2-stent strategy. Angiographic restenosis was more frequent in lesions with underexpansion than in lesions without underexpansion (24.1% vs 5.4%, respectively; P = .001), even in the 2-stent group (restenosis occurred in only 6% of those with complete expansion, compared with 6% in the single-stent group and 4.5% in nonbifurcation LMCA lesions). IVUS minimum stent area predicted angiographic restenosis 9 months after drug-eluting stent implantation and stent underexpansion was an independent predictor of repeat revascularization at 2 years.[28] However, although these minimal stent area values are useful for PCI guidance, every case needs to be individualized, particularly for different LMCA anatomic sizes; Fig. 13).

Assessment of the left circumflex ostium after provisional stenting

Lumen loss at the left circumflex ostium frequently occurs after crossover stenting from the distal LMCA into the left anterior descending

Preference for provisional stenting (1 stent)

- Small LCx
- No LCx disease
- Lesion in ostial LCx extending <5 mm
- No significant ostial LCx disease by IVUS (MLA >4 mm² and PB <50%)

Preference for 2-stent technique

No small LCx with any of the following:

- Significant and long (>5 mm) lesion in ostial LCx
- Complex lesion in ostial LCx
- Significant ostial LCx disease by IVUS (MLA <4 mm² and PB >50%)
- Poor result after provisional stenting:
  - Stenosis >75%
  - Reduced flow (TIMI flow <III)
  - Dissection
  - Ostial LCx with MLA less than 4 mm² after cross-over stenting

Abbreviations: IVUS, intravascular ultrasound; LCx, left circumflex; LMCA, left main coronary artery; MLA, minimal lumen area; PB, plaque burden; PCI, percutaneous coronary intervention; TIMI, thrombolysis in myocardial infarction.

(Fig. 14). The main mechanism involved is carina shift associated with a narrow angle between the left anterior descending and the left circumflex. In a study of 23 patients, the MLA of the ostial left circumflex decreased from 5.4 mm² before single-stent crossover to 4 mm² after stenting.[29] FFR can estimate better the functional impact of this lumen loss. However, if the residual MLA is greater than 3.5 to 4 mm², there are probably few, if any, repercussions. This is also true for restenosis risk (the most frequent reason for new revascularization in single-stent–treated distal LMCA lesions). As noted, a preprocedural MLA of the ostial left circumflex less than 3.7 mm² was strongly predictive of a post-stenting FFR of less than 0.80.[27] In sum, in LMCA bifurcation lesions with mild left circumflex ostial disease, the use of a single-stent technique rarely resulted in the functional left circumflex compromise and that because a functionally significant left circumflex stenosis is poorly predicted by a small MLA, side branch

treatment should be based on the post-stenting FFR.

IMPACT OF INTRAVASCULAR ULTRASOUND-GUIDED LEFT MAIN PERCUTANEOUS CORONARY INTERVENTION ON CLINICAL OUTCOMES

LMCA PCI is the treatment of choice in selected cases. The safety and efficacy of drug-eluting stents have enabled PCI outcomes to be similar to those of cardiac surgery, particularly when the extent and complexity of the coronary disease is not very high.

However, patients treated with drug-eluting stents from LMCA disease still suffer from restenosis and thrombosis, so the outcomes can continue to be improved. In the uniquely challenging anatomic scenario of the LMCA, the use of IVUS has been advocated as a means to optimize procedural results with the hope that this may translate into improved long-term clinical outcomes. The role of IVUS guidance in PCI of the left main has been controversial. Current US guidelines provide a class IIb recommendation for IVUS guidance during LMCA PCI, and has been upgraded to a class IIa recommendation in the recently released European guidelines.[30,31] The lack of specific randomized trials focused on answering this question implies that current evidence relies on observational analysis. In this regard, small registries initially reported conflicting results.[32,33] However, the conflicting results regarding the influence of IVUS on clinical outcomes can in part be explained by significant differences in patient and procedural characteristics between the studies.[34] A post hoc analysis of the MAIN-COMPARE study examined clinical outcomes in 145 well-matched pairs of patients with and without IVUS guidance during PCI with drug-eluting stents[35] and found that the 3-year incidence of total mortality was lower in the IVUS-guided group (4.7% vs 16%; P = .048) with survival curves diverging beyond the second year after PCI. The use of IVUS did not influence the incidence of myocardial infarction or target lesion revascularization. This study has several notable limitations. Baseline characteristics were favorable to the IVUS-guided arm. Despite elegant, rigorous, and exhaustive statistical adjustments using propensity score matching analyses, it remains possible that some unmeasured confounders could also be more favorable in the IVUS-guided arm, therefore explaining the better outcomes in these patients. This is relevant owing to the potential

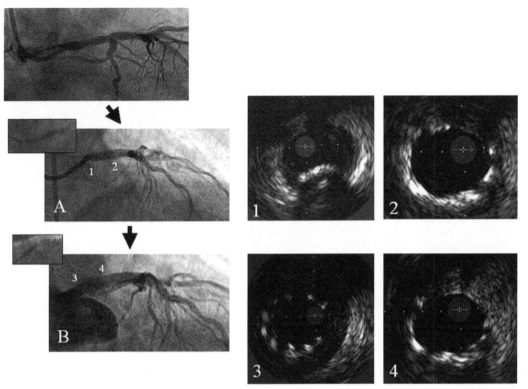

Fig. 11. Diffuse lesion in a long left main coronary artery treated with only angiographic guidance. (A) Angiographic result after stent implantation. Intravascular ultrasound shows noncovered LM ostium (1) and stent in the midshaft (2). (B) New short stent implanted at the ostial level (3) and first stent implanted in the midshaft (4).

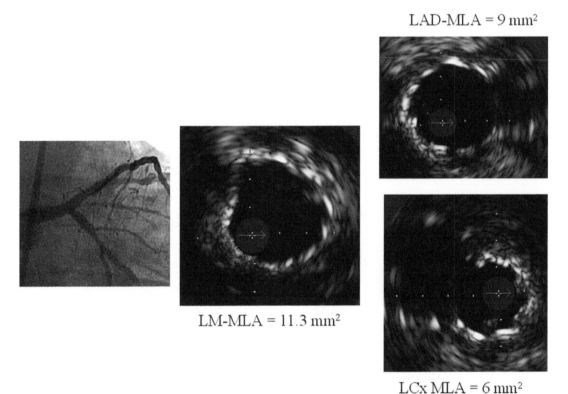

Fig. 12. Results after T-stenting technique of the distal left main bifurcation. LAD, left anterior descending; LCx, left circumflex; LM, left main; MLA, minimal lumen area.

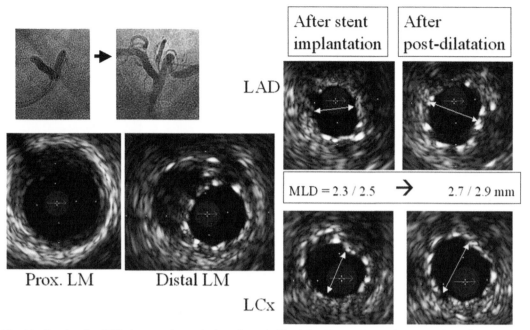

Fig. 13. Results after V/kissing stenting technique (case in **Fig. 10**) with two 3-mm diameter, drug-eluting stents and subsequent postdilatation with noncompliant balloons at 20 atm sequentially and with final kissing. The patient is an elderly woman with small body size. LAD, left anterior descending; LCx, left circumflex; LM, left main; MLD, minimal lumen diameter.

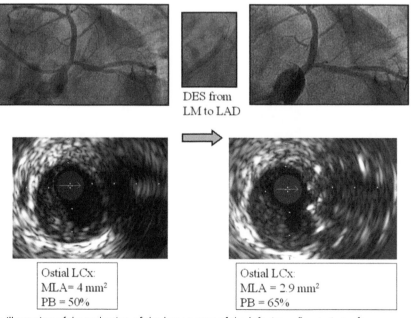

Fig. 14. Case illustration of the reduction of the lumen area of the left circumflex ostium after cross-over stenting from the left main coronary artery to the left anterior descending artery. LAD, left anterior descending; LCx, left circumflex; LM, left main; MLA, minimal lumen area; PB, plaque burden.

presence of severe noncardiac comorbidities, which are difficult to adjust for, in the cohort of complex patients who had angiographic guidance alone. Data regarding total mortality favoring IVUS guidance are difficult to interpret in the absence of comparative data on cardiac mortality and stent thrombosis. The very late effect of IVUS on survival is also intriguing.

More recently, in a multicenter study conducted by the ESTROFA (Grupo Español de Estudio de Stents Farmacoactivo) research group, which sought to compare the clinical outcomes of 770 patients treated with either first- or second-generation drug-eluting stents in the LMCA, the use of IVUS was found to be independent predictor of improved outcomes in the subgroup of patients with distal LMCA lesions.[36] Survival curves in the subgroup with distal lesions and in the subgroup with bifurcations treated with 2 stents showed wide and significant differences in death, myocardial infarction, and target lesion revascularization when stratified by IVUS use. In the multivariate analysis of the subgroup of patients with distal left main lesions, IVUS was an independent predictor for major adverse cardiac events, along with diabetes, age, and the use of 2 stents.

A total of 1670 patients with LMCA disease treated with drug-eluting stents were included in a pooled database of 4 registries, 2 of which were nationwide (ESTROFA-Left Main and RENACIMIENTO [Registro Nacional Sobre el Tratamiento del Tronco Común]) and 2 from single centers (Bellvitge and Valdecilla).[37] Among these, 505 patients (30.2%) underwent PCI of the LMCA under IVUS guidance (IVUS group). A second cohort of 505 patients treated without the use of IVUS during PCI was selected using propensity score matching (no IVUS group). Within the IVUS group, intravascular imaging was used to assess baseline lesion characteristics (plaque severity, extension, calcification, and ostial involvement) and then to guide PCI in 12% of patients. In the remaining 88% of cases, IVUS was used to guide PCI, allowing stent size selection after dilatation, assessment of stent coverage, expansion and apposition, and evaluation of side branch ostium when needed. Even though we included stent diameter and length in the propensity score matching process, diameters for main and side branch stents remained larger in the IVUS group than the no IVUS group. After IVUS examination, postdilatation (defined as dilatation with higher pressure and/or larger balloon) was done in a 40% of cases and a new stent was implanted

in 7.9% of patients. This information was not available for the angiogram-guided (no IVUS) group in all of the registries. In ESTROFA-Left Main and in the Valdecilla registry, post-dilatation in the IVUS-guided group was performed significantly more frequently and accomplished with larger balloons compared with angiography-guided PCI. Survival free of the combined endpoint of cardiac death, infarction, and target lesion revascularization was significantly better in the IVUS group. In addition, the incidence of definite and probable thrombosis was significantly lower in the IVUS group (0.6% vs 2.2%; $P = .04$). In the subgroup of patients with distal LMCA lesions, survival free of major adverse events (cardiac death, myocardial infarction, and target lesion revascularization) was significantly better for the IVUS group. Among those patients treated with 2 stents, the use of IVUS was associated with a significantly better outcome (**Fig. 15**). Notably, IVUS emerged as an independent predictor of fewer adverse events in the overall patient population and especially in the subgroup of patients with distal LMCA disease.[37]

TECHNICAL ISSUES IN THE INTRAVASCULAR ULTRASOUND ASSESSMENT OF THE LEFT MAIN CORONARY ARTERY

It is important to perform IVUS studies with enough quality to be able to obtain accurate and useful information. In the particular setting of the LMCA, the following techniques can be helpful.

Coaxial Guide Engagement
Attempt to get coaxial catheter alignment and disengage the catheter to assess properly the aorto–ostial junction. Examine the entire length of the LMCA up to the aorta, even in distal left main disease.

Manual Pullback
After an initial automatic pullback, it is often helpful to continue with a manual pullback to stop at the points of interest.

Intravascular Ultrasound Catheter Manipulation
Sometimes, owing to a marked angulation at the take-off of the left anterior descending or the left circumflex, the IVUS catheter may leap during either automatic or manual pullback, especially when the left circumflex ostium is highly calcified. This has been observed as well in LMCA ostial lesions. This prevents the proper

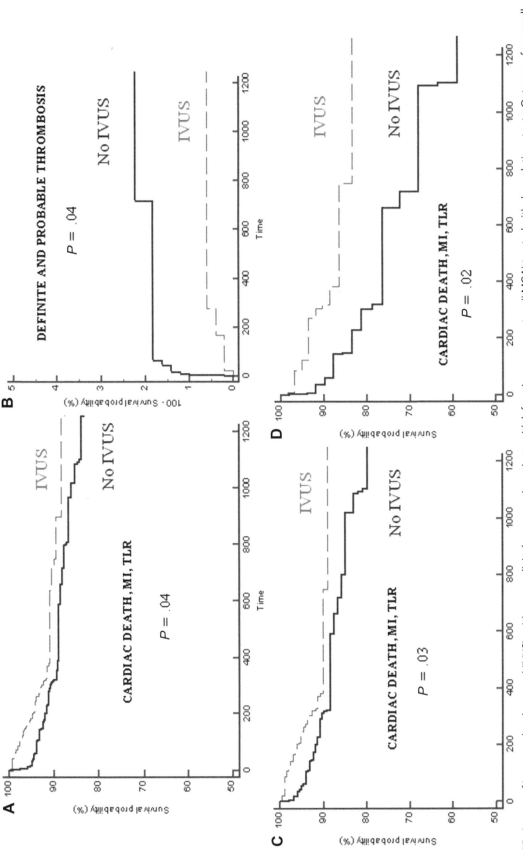

Fig. 15. Impact of intravascular ultrasound (IVUS) guidance on clinical outcomes in patients with left main coronary artery (LMCA) treated with drug-eluting stents. Outcomes for overall cohort. (A) Survival free of all-cause death, myocardial infarction and TLR. (B) Incidence of definite and probable thrombosis. Outcomes for the subgroups with (C) distal LMCA disease and (D) distal LMCA disease treated with 2 stents. MI, myocardial infarction; TLR, target lesion revascularization. (From De la Torre Hernandez JM, Baz JA, Gómez Hospital JA, et al. Clinical impact of intravascular ultrasound guidance in drug-eluting stent implantation for unprotected left main coronary disease: patient level pooled analysis of 4 registries. JACC Cardiovasc Interv 2014;7:250–2; with permission.)

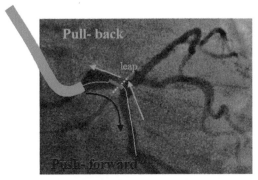

Fig. 16. The presence of intravascular ultrasound catheter leap during pullback imaging can be avoided with a gentle push-forward imaging.

assessment of the entire LMCA and, thus, the most critical MLA site can be missed. To avoid this problem, it is possible to perform a gentle manual push forward to image the area of interest. In our experience, with this maneuver a complete imaging of the entire LMCA can be obtained (Fig. 16).

Perform a Pullback from Both the Left Anterior Descending and Left Circumflex Arteries
It is important to assess the LMCA disease with distal involvement from both the left anterior

descending and left circumflex because the measurement of the MLA and the plaque burden of a side branch ostium a main vessel pullback is not accurate (it tends to overestimate the MLA owing to obliquity; Fig. 17). The "oblique view" detection of any plaque in the side branch predicted plaque burden with good sensitivity but poor specificity. IVUS evaluation of a side branch ostium from the main vessel is only moderately reliable, especially for distal LMCA lesions. For an accurate assessment of the side branch ostium, direct imaging is necessary.[38] In addition, the MLA of the LMCA differed by 1 mm^2 in 25% of patients when imaged from a pullback beginning in the LAD compared with a pullback beginning in the LCx. Because IVUS can increase artificially, but not decrease, lumen dimensions, the smallest MLA is always the most accurate.

Do No Harm
If the angle at the exit of a branch is pronounced (particularly the left circumflex) and the presence of calcium is significant, advancing the IVUS catheter advance can be difficult, so, to avoid iatrogenic dissections, excessive force should not be used.

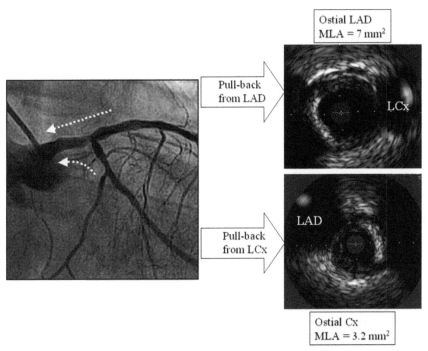

Fig. 17. It is important to assess the left main coronary artery disease with distal involvement from both branches because the measurement of the MLA and the plaque burden of a vessel from the complementary vessel pullback is inaccurate. LAD, left anterior descending; LCx, left circumflex; MLA, minimal lumen area.

SUMMARY

IVUS is helpful in the assessment of LMCA lesion severity, overcoming the multiple limitations of angiography within this anatomic segment. IVUS provides precise and detailed information regarding the atherosclerotic burden, plaque extension, and plaque morphology from the aorto–ostial junction to the distal segment and both the ostia of both the left anterior descending and left circumflex arteries. This information, along with other clinical data, can provide guidance with regard to the need for revascularization or deferral based on minimal luminal area. Furthermore, IVUS can be a useful tool to plan the PCI strategy and to optimize the results with respect to stent size, lesion coverage, stent apposition, expansion, and the detection of edge dissection. Observational studies have shown that IVUS guidance of LMCA PCI with drug-eluting stents improves clinical outcomes, particularly for the treatment of distal left main disease.

REFERENCES

1. Cameron A, Kemp HG Jr, Fisher LD, et al. Left main coronary artery stenosis: angiographic determination. Circulation 1983;68:484–9.
2. Fisher LD, Judkins MP, Lesperance J, et al. Reproducibility of coronary arteriographic reading in the Coronary Artery Study (CASS). Cathet Cardiovasc Diagn 1982;8:565–75.
3. Arnett EN, Isner JM, Redwood DR. Coronary artery narrowing in coronary heart disease: comparison of cineangiographic and necropsy findings. Ann Intern Med 1979;91:350–6.
4. Isner JM, Kishel J, Kent KM, et al. Accuracy of angiographic determination of left main coronary arterial narrowing. Angiographic–histologic correlative analysis in 28 patients. Circulation 1981;63:1056–64.
5. Hermiller JB, Buller CE, Tenaglia AN, et al. Unrecognized left main coronary artery disease in patients undergoing interventional procedures. Am J Cardiol 1993;71:173–6.
6. Gerber TC, Erbel R, Gorge G, et al. Extent of atherosclerosis and remodeling of the left main coronary artery determined by intravascular ultrasound. Am J Cardiol 1994;73:666–71.
7. Wolfhard U, Gorge G, Konorza T, et al. Intravascular ultrasound examination reverses therapeutic decision from percutaneous intervention to a surgical approach in patients with alterations of the left main stem. Thorac Cardiovasc Surg 1998;5:281–4.
8. Abizaid AS, Mintz GS, Abizaid A, et al. One-year follow-up after intravascular ultrasound assessment of moderate left main coronary artery disease in patients with ambiguous angiograms. J Am Coll Cardiol 1999;34:707–15.
9. Ricciardi MJ, Meyers S, Choi K, et al. Angiographically silent left main disease detected by intravascular ultrasound: a marker for future adverse cardiac events. Am Heart J 2003;146:507–12.
10. Jasti V, Ivan E, Yalamanchili V, et al. Correlations between fractional flow reserve and intravascular ultrasound in patients with an ambiguous left main coronary artery stenosis. Circulation 2004;110:2831–6.
11. Park SJ, Ahn JM, Kang SJ, et al. Intravascular ultrasound-derived minimal lumen area criteria for functionally significant left main coronary artery stenosis. JACC Cardiovasc Interv 2014;7:868–74.
12. Nascimento BR, de Sousa MR, Koo BK, et al. Diagnostic accuracy of intravascular ultrasound-derived minimal lumen area compared with fractional flow reserve meta-analysis: pooled accuracy of IVUS luminal area versus FFR. Catheter Cardiovasc Interv 2014;84:377–85.
13. Fassa AA, Wagatsuma K, Higano ST, et al. Intravascular ultrasound-guided treatment for angiographically indeterminate left main coronary artery disease: a long-term follow-up study. J Am Coll Cardiol 2005;45:204–11.
14. Finet G, Gilard M, Perrenot B, et al. Fractal geometry of arterial coronary bifurcations: a quantitative coronary angiography and intravascular ultrasound analysis. EuroIntervention 2008;3:490–8.
15. Huo Y, Finet G, Lefèvre T, et al. Optimal diameter of diseased bifurcation segment: a practical rule for percutaneous coronary intervention. EuroIntervention 2012;7:1310–6.
16. De la Torre Hernandez JM, Hernandez Hernandez F, Alfonso F, et al. Prospective application of pre-defined intravascular ultrasound criteria for assessment of intermediate left main coronary artery lesions results from the multicenter LITRO study. J Am Coll Cardiol 2011;58:351–8.
17. De la Torre Hernandez JM, Ruiz Lera M, Fernandez Friera L, et al. Prospective use of an intravascular ultrasound-derived minimum lumen area cut-off value in the assessment of intermediate left main coronary artery lesions. Rev Esp Cardiol 2007;60:811–6.
18. Lee DH, Arnaez Corada B, De la Torre Hernández JM, et al. Safety in a very long term follow-up (> 5 years) of a cut-off value of 6 mm^2 for the minimum lumen area of intermediate left main coronary artery lesions. Am J Cardiol 2013;111(7S):41B.
19. Rusinova RP, Mintz GS, Choi SY, et al. Intravascular ultrasound comparison of left main coronary artery disease between white and Asian patients. Am J Cardiol 2013;111:979–84.

20. Waksman R, Legutko J, Singh J, et al. FIRST: fractional flow reserve and intravascular ultrasound relationship study. J Am Coll Cardiol 2013;61: 917–23.

21. Okabe T, Mintz GS, Lee SY, et al. Five-year outcomes of moderate or ambiguous left main coronary artery disease and the intravascular ultrasound predictors of events. J Invasive Cardiol 2008;20:635–9.

22. Yong AS, Daniels D, De Bruyne B, et al. Fractional flow reserve assessment of left main stenosis in the presence of downstream coronary stenoses. Circ Cardiovasc Interv 2013;6:161–5.

23. Maehara A, Mintz GS, Castagna MT, et al. Intravascular ultrasound assessment of the stenoses location and morphology in the left main coronary artery in relation to anatomic left main length. Am J Cardiol 2001;88:1–4.

24. Oviedo C, Maehara A, Mintz GS, et al. Intravascular ultrasound classification of plaque distribution in left main coronary artery bifurcations: where is the plaque really located? Circ Cardiovasc Interv 2010;3:105–12.

25. Valgimigli M, Rodriguez-Granillo GA, Garcia-Garcia HM, et al. Plaque composition in the left main stem mimics the distal but not the proximal tract of the left coronary artery: influence of clinical presentation, length of the left main trunk, lipid profile, and systemic levels of C-reactive protein. J Am Coll Cardiol 2007;49:23–31.

26. Mercado N, Moe TG, Pieper M, et al. Tissue characterisation of atherosclerotic plaque in the left main: an in vivo intravascular ultrasound radiofrequency data analysis. EuroIntervention 2011;7: 347–52.

27. Kang SJ, Ahn JM, Kim WJ, et al. Functional and morphological assessment of side branch after left main coronary artery bifurcation stenting with cross-over technique. Catheter Cardiovasc Interv 2014;83:545–52.

28. Kang SJ, Ahn JM, Song H, et al. Comprehensive intravascular ultrasound assessment of stent area and its impact on restenosis and adverse cardiac events in 403 patients with unprotected left main disease. Circ Cardiovasc Interv 2011;4:562–9.

29. Kang SJ, Mintz GS, Kim WJ, et al. Changes in left main bifurcation geometry after a single-stent crossover technique: an intravascular ultrasound study using direct imaging of both the left anterior descending and the left circumflex coronary arteries before and after intervention. Circ Cardiovasc Interv 2011;4:355–61.

30. Levine GN, Bates ER, Blankenship JC, et al. 2011 ACCF/AHA/SCAI guideline for percutaneous coronary intervention: a report of the American college of cardiology foundation/American heart association task force on practice guidelines and the society for cardiovascular angiography and interventions. J Am Coll Cardiol 2011;58:e44–122.

31. Windecker S, Kolh P, Alfonso F, et al. 2014 ESC/EACTS guidelines on myocardial revascularization: the task force on myocardial revascularization of the European society of cardiology (ESC) and the European association for cardio-thoracic surgery (EACTS)developed with the special contribution of the European association of percutaneous cardiovascular interventions (EAPCI). Eur Heart J 2014;35:2541–619.

32. Agostoni P, Valgimigli M, Van Mieghem CA, et al. Comparison of early outcome of percutaneous coronary intervention for unprotected left main coronary artery disease in the drug-eluting stent era with versus without intravascular ultrasonic guidance. Am J Cardiol 2005;95:644–7.

33. Park SJ, Kim YH, Lee BK, et al. Sirolimus-eluting stent implantation for unprotected left main coronary artery stenosis: comparison with bare metal stent implantation. J Am Coll Cardiol 2005;45:351–6.

34. Park DW, Kim YH, Yun SC, et al. Long-term outcomes after stenting versus coronary artery bypass grafting for unprotected left main coronary artery disease: 10-year results of bare-metal stents and 5-year results of drug-eluting stents from the ASAN-MAIN (ASAN Medical Center-Left MAIN Revascularization) registry. J Am Coll Cardiol 2010;56:1366–75.

35. Park SJ, Kim YH, Park DW, et al. MAIN-COMPARE investigators. Impact of intravascular ultrasound guidance on long-term mortality in stenting for unprotected left main coronary artery stenosis. Circ Cardiovasc Interv 2009;2:167–77.

36. De la Torre Hernandez JM, Alfonso F, Recalde AS, et al. Comparison of paclitaxel-eluting stents (Taxus) and everolimus-eluting stents (Xience) in left main coronary artery disease with 3 years follow-up (from the ESTROFA-LM registry). Am J Cardiol 2013;111:676–83.

37. De la Torre Hernandez JM, Baz JA, Gómez Hospital JA, et al. Clinical impact of intravascular ultrasound guidance in drug-eluting stent implantation for unprotected left main coronary disease: patient level pooled analysis of 4 registries. JACC Cardiovasc Interv 2014;7:244–54.

38. Oviedo C, Maehara A, Mintz GS, et al. Is accurate intravascular ultrasound evaluation of the left circumflex ostium from a left anterior descending to left main pullback possible? Am J Cardiol 2010;105:948–54.

Intravascular Ultrasound for the Assessment of Coronary Lesion Severity and Optimization of Percutaneous Coronary Interventions

Seung-Jung Park, MD, PhD*, Jung-Min Ahn, MD

KEYWORDS

- Intravascular ultrasound • Coronary disease • Stent

KEY POINTS

- The major use of intravascular ultrasound (IVUS) is to plan interventional strategy and optimize stent deployment.
- The use of IVUS to identify which lesions should be treated is problematic: recent data suggest that a minimal lumen area (MLA) ≤ 2.4 mm^2 may be the optimal cutoff to predict functional significance by fractional flow reserve, although IVUS-derived MLA alone cannot replace noninvasive or invasive functional assessment.
- Stent optimization by IVUS includes the evaluation of stent expansion, apposition, lesion coverage, and the presence or absence of stent edge dissection.
- Observational studies suggest that IVUS guidance during drug-eluting stent implantation reduces the risk of major adverse cardiac events, including stent thrombosis, particularly in the setting of unprotected left main percutaneous coronary interventions (PCI).
- The as-treated analysis of the long-lesion RESET randomized trial reported that the use of IVUS guidance during PCI with a drug-eluting stent resulted in significantly larger final minimal stent area and a lower risk of 1-year major adverse cardiac events compared with angiographic guidance alone.

INTRODUCTION

Intravascular ultrasound (IVUS) has provided valuable information regarding cross-sectional coronary vascular structure (Fig. 1). It plays a key role in contemporary stent-based percutaneous coronary interventions (PCI) by accurately assessing coronary anatomy, assisting in selection of treatment strategy, and defining optimal stenting outcomes.[1–3] In the bare metal stent (BMS) era, randomized trials and meta-analyses reported that IVUS-guided PCI was associated with a lower risk of angiographic restenosis and target vessel revascularization than PCI guided by angiography alone.[4,5] Drug-eluting stents (DES), which markedly reduce the rate of in-stent restenosis and target vessel revascularization, could therefore reduce the clinical usefulness of IVUS. However, the reduced risk of in-stent restenosis with DES is offset by concerns about stent thrombosis. In addition, the increased use of DES has led to the treatment

---

The authors have nothing to disclose.
Division of Cardiology, Asan Medical Center, University of Ulsan College of Medicine, 388-1, Poongnap-dong, Songpa-gu, Seoul 138-736, South Korea
* Corresponding author.
E-mail address: sjpark@amc.seoul.kr

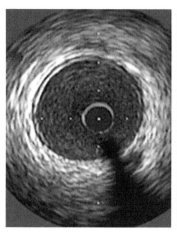
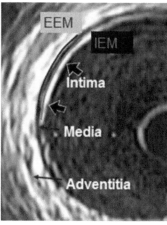

Fig. 1. IVUS findings of normal coronary artery. EEM, external elastic membrane; IEM, internal elastic membrane.

of more complex lesions and higher-risk patients, in which the risk of early and late stent failure is greater. A recent meta-analysis[6] reported the benefit of IVUS-guided DES implantation compared with angiography-guided implantation in reducing the risk of death, myocardial infarction, stent thrombosis, and repeat revascularization. In this review, a comprehensive approach to the evaluation of coronary lesions and the optimization of PCI with DES using IVUS is presented.

INTRAVASCULAR LESION ASSESSMENT
Anatomic Lesion Assessment
The major use for IVUS is to plan interventional strategy and optimize stent deployment. Preintervention IVUS accurately assesses reference lumen dimensions and lesion length for appropriate stent sizing (Fig. 2). In addition, IVUS

findings such as severe superficial calcium, or thrombus, can alter the mechanical or pharmacologic strategy, including prestent rotational atherectomy for plaque modification, more potent anticoagulant therapies, or mechanical thrombectomy. Poststent IVUS assessment may detect complications of PCI and suboptimal stent deployment (Fig. 3),[7] which lead to further interventions for optimal stent implantation, thereby minimizing stent-related adverse clinical outcomes. Table 1 summarizes the quantitative and qualitative parameters measured by IVUS before and after stent implantation.[1]

Functional Lesion Assessment
Although IVUS cannot directly estimate the functional significance of coronary stenosis, attempts have been made to determine the IVUS parameters that correspond to a functionally significant

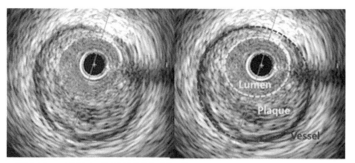
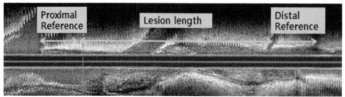

Fig. 2. IVUS evaluation of diseased lesion.

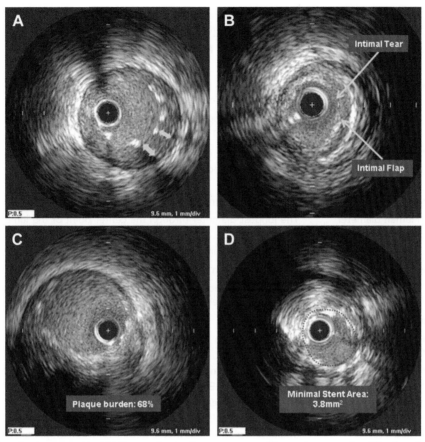

Fig. 3. Suboptimal stent results of (*A*) acute incomplete stent apposition underexpansion, (*B*) edge dissection, (*C*) large edge plaque burden, (*D*) underexpansion.

coronary artery narrowing, thus integrating target lesion anatomy and physiology (Table 2). Over the last 10 years, many interventionists have used the threshold of minimal lumen area (MLA) less than 4 mm^2 on IVUS to identify lesions that require stent implantation. However, Kang and colleagues[8] evaluated 201 patients with 236 coronary lesions who underwent preintervention IVUS and fractional flow reserve (FFR) measurements to determine the best IVUS MLA criteria corresponding to FFR less than 0.80. These investigators reported that the optimal cutoff value of IVUS MLA for predicting FFR less than 0.80 (ie, providing the greatest sum of sensitivity and specificity) was less than 2.4 mm^2, a figure substantially smaller than previously reported. In addition, despite this strict criterion, the positive predictive value of IVUS to predict functional significance was poor. Therefore, IVUS-derived MLA alone cannot replace the role of noninvasive or invasive functional studies in making clinical decisions about whether to dilate a coronary stenosis that does not involve the left main.[8–16]

STENT OPTIMIZATION
Limitations of Compliance Chart-Dependent Stenting
Visual estimation or even quantitative angiographic analyses of vessel dimension for stent deployment seem inaccurate.[17–19] In addition, angiographic success cannot always be linked with optimal stent expansion, even with higher-pressure balloon inflation during the stenting procedure. The achievement of optimal stent deployment by IVUS with normal-to-high pressure balloon dilation was evaluated in 256 patients undergoing BMS implantation. Only 14% of patients achieved optimal stent deployment with dilations under 12-atm pressures, and only 36% of cases achieved optimal deployment even with higher deployment pressures (>14 atm).[18] In another study with an early-generation DES, stent expansion was assessed by IVUS in 200 patients using the manufacturer's compliance chart as a reference. According to IVUS, the DES achieved only 75% of the predicted minimal stent diameter and 66% of the predicted minimal stent area (MSA).[19]

Table 1
Quantitative and qualitative IVUS measurement

Quantitative Measurement

Reference and stenotic lesion

Reference (proximal or distal)	The site with the largest lumen proximal or distal to a stenosis but within the same segment (<10 mm)
Stenosis	A lesion that compromises the lumen by >50% by cross-sectional area compared with a reference segment lumen

Lumen measurement

Lumen cross-sectional area (CSA)	The area bounded by the luminal border
Minimum lumen diameter	The shortest diameter through the center point of the lumen
Maximum lumen diameter	The longest diameter through the center point of the lumen
Lumen eccentricity	(Maximum lumen diameter–minimum lumen diameter)/maximum lumen diameter
Lumen area stenosis	(Reference lumen CSA–minimum lumen CSA)/reference lumen CSA
External elastic membrane (EEM) CSA	EEM is an interface at the border between the media and the adventitia. Alternative terms: vessel area, total vessel area

Atheroma measurement

Plaque + media CSA (atheroma area)	EEM CSA–lumen CSA
Maximum plaque + media (or atheroma) thickness	The largest distance from the intimal leading edge to the EEM along any line passing through the center of the lumen
Minimum plaque + media (or atheroma) thickness	The shortest distance from intimal leading edge to the EEM along any line passing through the luminal center of mass
Plaque + media (or atheroma) eccentricity	(Maximum plaque plus media thickness–minimum plaque plus media thickness)/maximum plaque plus media thickness
Plaque (or atheroma) burden	Plaque + media CSA/EEM CSA

Calcium measurement

Superficial/deep calcium	The leading edge of the acoustic shadowing appears within the most shallow/the deepest 50% of the plaque plus media thickness
Arc	Measured in degrees by using an electronic protractor centered on the lumen
Semiquantitation	Absent or subtending 1, 2, 3, or 4 quadrants

Stent measurement

Stent CSA	The area bounded by the stent border
Minimum stent diameter	The shortest diameter through the center of mass of the stent
Maximum stent diameter	The longest diameter through the center of mass of the stent
Stent symmetry	(Maximum stent diameter–minimum stent diameter)/maximum stent diameter
Vascular remodeling	Lesion EEM CSA/reference EEM CSA. If index >1.0, positive remodeling; if index <1.0, negative remodeling

Qualitative Measurement

Soft (echolucent) plaques	The acoustic signal that arises from low echogenicity. This is generally the result of high lipid content in a mostly cellular lesion
Fibrous plaques	These plaques have an intermediate echogenicity between soft atheroma and highly echogenic calcific plaque

(continued on next page)

Table 1 (continued)	
Qualitative Measurement	
Attenuated plaques	These plaques have the absence of the ultrasound signal behind plaque that was either hypoechoic or isoechoic to the reference adventitia but contained no echoes that were brighter than the adventitia
Calcified nodules	Distinct calcification with an irregular, protruding, and convex luminal surface
Thrombus	Usually recognized as an intraluminal mass, often with a layered, lobulated, or pedunculated appearance. Thrombi may appear relatively echolucent or have more variable gray scale, with speckling or scintillation
Intimal hyperplasia	Characteristic of early in-stent restenosis often appears as low echogenicity, at times less echogenic than the blood speckle in the lumen. The intimal hyperplasia of late in-stent restenosis often appears more echogenic
Plaque ulceration	A recess in the plaque beginning at the luminal-intimal border, typically without enlargement of the EEM compared with the reference segment
Plaque rupture	A plaque ulceration with a tear detected in a fibrous cap (contrast injections may be used to prove and define the communication point)
True aneurysm	A lesion that includes all the layers of the vessel wall with an EEM and lumen area 50% larger than the proximal reference segment
Pseudoaneurysm	A maximum lumen area >50% larger than proximal reference lumen area with loss of vessel wall integrity
Stent fracture	Stent fracture was defined as absence of all stent struts in ≥ 1 cross section
Incomplete stent apposition	A lack of contact between stent struts and the underlying vessel wall not overlying a side branch

Therefore, simply using the manufacturer's compliance chart to predict the resulting stent diameter after deployment is frequently inaccurate and may lead to substantial stent undersizing and underexpansion. Adequate postdeployment stent evaluation by IVUS may therefore be important to obtain optimal stent expansion as well as improve short-term and long-term clinical outcomes.

Minimal Stent Cross-Sectional Area

The concept of the bigger the better is still valid in the DES era. Proper stent expansion is essential to prevent DES stent thrombosis as well as restenosis at follow-up.[20,21] Serial IVUS analysis from the SIRIUS (Sirolimus-Eluting Stent in Coronary Lesions) trial[22] indicated that an MSA less than 5.0 mm^2 was associated with most cases of restenosis. Similarly, Hong and colleagues[23] found in a large series of patients treated with sirolimus-eluting stent implantation that an MSA of 5.5 mm^2 best separated cases with

subsequent in-stent restenosis from those without restenosis. Another study using paclitaxel-eluting stents[24] identified an MSA ≥ 5.7 mm^2 as the best cutoff associated with a reduced risk of 9-month in-stent restenosis. Examination of sensitivity and specificity curves in these 3 analyses confirmed that the MSA that best separated cases with first-generation DES restenosis from without restenosis was between 5.0 and 6.0 mm^2. However, an MSA greater than 5.0 mm^2 may not be achievable in small vessels; in these cases, stent expansion represented as MSA/reference lumen may be a predictor of an adequate lumen at follow-up.[25] Song and colleagues[26] explored the optimal postimplantation MSA for second-generation DES by identifying the best cutoff value to predict 9-month in-stent restenosis in 220 zotarolimus-eluting stents and 229 everolimus-eluting stents. For zotarolimus-eluting stents, the optimal MSA predicting in-stent restenosis was 5.3 mm^2, and for the everolimus-eluting stent, an MSA less

Table 2
IVUS-measured MLA criteria for functionally significant lesions

	Nishioka et al,[9] 1999	Briguori et al,[10] 2001	Takagi et al,[11] 1999	Abizaid et al,[12] 1998	Kang et al,[8] 2011	Kang et al,[13] 2012	Ben-Dor et al,[14] 2012	Koo et al,[15] 2011	Gonzalo et al,[16] 2012
Functional study	Thallium(+)	FFR<0.75	FFR<0.75	CFR≥2.0	FFR<0.8	FFR<0.8	FFR<0.8	FFR<0.8	FFR<0.8
Lesion number (n)	70	53	51	112	236	784	205	267	47
Cutoff MLA (mm^2)	≤4.0	≤4.0	<3.0	≥4.0	<2.4	<2.4	<3.09	<2.75	<2.36
Accuracy (%)	NA	79	90.2	89	68	69	70	67	66
Sensitivity (%)	90	92	83.0	NA	90	84	69	69	67
Specificity (%)	88	56	92.3	NA	60	63	72	65	65

Abbreviation: FFR, fractional flow reserve.

than 5.4 mm^2 predicted in-stent restenosis, similar to that observed with first-generation DES. Several studies have also reported that an MSA less than 5 mm^2 is associated with stent thrombosis.[20,21,27]

Stent Edge Plaque Burden

Residual plaque burden is also a predictor of late stent thrombosis and edge restenosis. Fujii and colleagues[20] reported that the presence of a significant residual reference segment stenosis (defined as edge lumen cross-sectional area <4 mm^2 and a plaque burden >70%) was more common in cases of stent thrombosis compared with a matched control group (67% vs 9%, P<.001). In addition, a significant residual reference segment stenosis was identified as an independent predictor of stent thrombosis (P = .02). Consistently, Okabe and colleagues[21] reported that patients with DES who developed stent thrombosis had a smaller MSA and more residual disease at the stent edges, with a larger plaque burden. In the SIRIUS trial, a larger percentage plaque area at the reference segment was associated with edge restenosis, indicating that inadequate lesion coverage may contribute to edge stenosis and target lesion revascularization.[28] To confirm full lesion coverage and a proper match between the stented and adjacent segments, use of IVUS may improve outcomes in patients receiving DES implantation.

Stent Length

The relative impact of the final MSA and stent length on the incidence of restenosis were reduced in the DES era because of the profound antiproliferative effect of the eluted drug. However, an IVUS-measured stent length greater than 40 mm predicted 6-month angiographic restenosis after sirolimus-eluting stent implantation with a sensitivity of 81% and a specificity of 78%.[23] In addition, a stent length threshold of 31.5 mm predicted the incidence of stent thrombosis with a sensitivity and specificity of 88.4% and 52.1%, respectively. Stent lengths ≥31.5 mm were associated with higher rates of stent thrombosis (4.0% vs 0.7%, P<.001), death (5.2% vs 3.0%, P = .005), and myocardial infarction (2.4% vs 0.7%, P = .001) at 3 years, compared with stent lengths less than 31.5 mm.[29]

However, IVUS utilization may attenuate the detrimental effect of the increase of implanted stent length, particularly during PCI with long stent implantation.[30] IVUS examinations can detect such mechanical factors earlier and more frequently prompt further interventions for optimal stent implantation, thereby minimizing stent-related adverse clinical outcomes associated with increased implanted stent length. Ahn and colleagues[30] reported that when IVUS was used during PCI, clinical outcomes at 2 years were not significantly different according to the implanted stent length (**Fig. 4**A). However, without IVUS use, as the length of stents increased, the rate of adverse events also increased (see **Fig. 4**B). Therefore, when long stent implantation is attempted, physicians should consider IVUS examinations to reduce the rate of adverse events.

Stent Edge Dissection

Stent edge dissection is associated with large or asymmetric residual plaque burden, calcified plaque, or implantation of a relatively large diameter stent. Significant edge dissection,

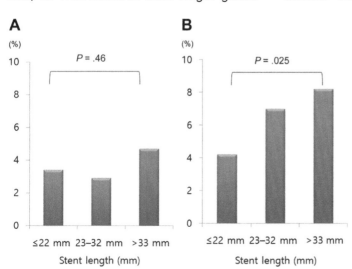

A

B

Fig. 4. The occurrence of death, myocardial infarction, or target vessel revascularization according to implanted stent length and IVUS use. (A) IVUS use; (B) no IVUS use. (*Data from* Ahn JM, Han S, Park YK, et al. Differential prognostic effect of intravascular ultrasound use according to implanted stent length. Am J Cardiol 2013;111:829–35.)

defined as lumen narrowing less than 4 mm^2 or dissection angle $\geq 60°$, has been associated with an increased incidence of early stent thrombosis; thus, additional stents may be needed to prevent stent thrombosis.[31] However, a minor dissection, detected by IVUS, may not be associated with an increased incidence of stent thrombosis.[32,33] Although no consensus exists on an optimal strategy, in the presence of minor dissection, careful observation without stenting might be considered.[34]

Incomplete Stent Apposition

Incomplete stent apposition (ISA) is defined as the absence of contact between the stent struts and the lumen wall and can occur acutely after stent deployment (acute ISA) or develop over time (late-acquired ISA). Most acute ISA resolves over time and does not affect the incidence of stent thrombosis or in-stent restenosis. Hong and colleagues[35] showed that postprocedure ISA occurred in 7.2% of DES-treated lesions and was not associated with major adverse cardiac events, including target lesion revascularization or even an increased amount of intimal hyperplasia. In the TAXUS-II trial, 8 of 13 cases of acute ISA in the slow-release group resolved, all acute ISA in the moderate-release group resolved, and at 12 months, acute ISA was not associated with an increase in adverse clinical events.[36] In addition, In the HORIZONS-AMI (Harmonizing Outcomes with Revascularization and Stents in Acute Myocardial Infarction) trial, although acute ISA was detected in 33.8% of 68 lesions treated with a paclitaxel-eluting stent, there was no difference in the rate of major adverse cardiac events in patients with acute ISA compared with those without acute ISA.[37] Therefore, because of the lack of evidence of a relationship between acute ISA and adverse cardiac events, overly aggressive additional inflations to eliminate acute ISA seem unwarranted.

The mechanism for late-acquired ISA is different from acute ISA and is believed to be related to positive remodeling of the vessel, resolution of thrombus present at the time of the initial stent deployment, or a delayed-type hypersensitivity reaction.[7] In addition, the risk of stent thrombosis-related late ISA is unclear. Cook and colleagues[38] showed that the rate of late ISA was significantly higher in patients with DES thrombosis than in control patients without stent thrombosis (77% vs 12%, P<.001). However, in a pooled study of 1580 patients enrolled in the IVUS substudies of multiple TAXUS stent trials, there were 36 cases of late-acquired ISA

at 9-month follow-up, which were not associated with increased rates of stent thrombosis or major adverse cardiac events over the ensuing 2 years.[39]

Box 1 summarizes the criteria for optimal stent deployment, including complete stent apposition to the vessel wall, adequate stent expansion, and full lesion coverage without edge dissection.

INTRAVASCULAR ULTRASOUND–GUIDED PERCUTANEOUS CORONARY INTERVENTION: CLINICAL DATA

Observational Studies

Several nonrandomized, observational studies have examined the impact of IVUS guidance on clinical outcomes after PCI with DES. In a study of unselected 884 propensity-matched patients, IVUS-guided DES implantation was found to significantly reduce the rates of definite stent thrombosis at 30 days and 12 months. The IVUS-guided group showed significant reductions in definite subacute stent thrombosis (0.5% vs 1.4%, $P = .045$) and cumulative stent thrombosis (0.7% vs 2.0%, $P = .014$) at 12 months compared with the angiography-guided group.[40] Another large real-world registry from 2 Korean centers reported long-term outcomes of both IVUS- and angiography-guided PCI using DES implantation. In patients receiving DES, the 3-year adjusted incidence of mortality was significantly lower in the IVUS-guided PCI group compared with the angiography-guided PCI group (hazard ratio [HR], 0.70; 95% confidence interval [CI], 0.56–0.87; $P = .001$). However, IVUS-guided PCI did not influence the rates of myocardial infarction, target vessel revascularization, or stent thrombosis.[41] The IVUS substudy of the ADAPT-DES (Platelet Reactivity and Clinical Outcomes After Coronary Artery Implantation of Drug-Eluting Stents) study is one of the largest observational studies yet performed to assess the influence of IVUS guidance on clinical outcomes. In this

---

Box 1
Criteria for optimal stent deployment

- Complete stent apposition to the vessel wall
- Adequate stent expansion (ie, >MSA of 5.0–5.5 mm^2)
- Full lesion coverage with minimal residual plaque burden
- No stent-related complications (such as edge dissection, stent fracture, thrombus, or others)

study, a total of 8583 patients were enrolled (IVUS-guided PCI in 3349 patients and angiography-guided PCI in 5234 patients).[42] IVUS guidance changed the procedural approach in about 75% of cases, such as the selection of a larger stent or balloon size, after dilatation, additional stent implantation, or the use of higher-pressure inflations. At 1-year follow-up, IVUS guidance was associated with a lower rate of stent thrombosis, myocardial infarction, and target lesion revascularization.

Routine IVUS examination may be particularly useful during PCI of certain anatomic subsets, such as left main coronary artery disease, bifurcation disease, and long lesions. At 4-year follow-up, IVUS-guided DES implantation for bifurcation lesions significantly reduced the rates of mortality and very late stent thrombosis compared with conventional angiography-guided stenting.[43] In addition, the use of IVUS reduced the risk of side branch occlusion after main vessel stenting.[44] In the MAIN-COMPARE (Revascularization for Unprotected Left Main Coronary Artery Stenosis: Comparison of Percutaneous Coronary Angioplasty Versus Surgical Revascularization) registry, patients with unprotected left main coronary artery stenosis in a hemodynamically stable condition underwent elective stenting under the guidance of IVUS (756 patients) or conventional angiography (219 patients). In 145 matched pairs of patients receiving DES, the 3-year incidence of mortality was significantly lower with IVUS guidance compared with angiographic guidance (4.7% vs 16.0%, log-rank $P = .048$; HR, 0.39). Another study that examined outcomes among 505 propensity score-matched pairs undergoing unprotected left main PCI with DES also reported that IVUS guidance was associated with a reduced risk of death or stent thrombosis.[45]

Randomized Studies
To date, 3 randomized studies have investigated the clinical efficacy of an IVUS-guided strategy in PCI with DES. The HOME-DES (Long-Term Health Outcome and Mortality Evaluation After Invasive Coronary Treatment Using Drug Eluting Stents With or Without the IVUS Guidance) study randomly assigned 210 patients to either an IVUS-guided PCI strategy or an angiography-guided strategy.[46] The IVUS-guided strategy led to more frequent postdilations, higher balloon inflation pressures, and larger balloon sizes, but it did not result in an improvement in clinical outcomes. In the AVIO (Angiography vs IVUS Optimization) trial, IVUS guidance led to

larger stent dimensions, but this did not translate into improved clinical outcomes at 9-month follow-up. Both HOME-DES and AVIO are limited by a relatively short follow-up period and are statistical underpowered to detect significant differences in clinical outcomes.[47]

The prespecified long-lesion subset from the RESET (Real Safety and Efficacy of a 3-Month Dual Antiplatelet Therapy Following Zotarolimus-Eluting Stents Implantation) trial is the only randomized study powered to detect an influence of IVUS on clinical outcomes.[14] In this study, 543 patients were randomly assigned to either IVUS-guided or angiography-guided implantation of long ($\geq$28 mm) DES. In the intention-to-treat analysis of this trial, IVUS-guided PCI was not associated with a significant reduction in major adverse cardiac events, defined as a composite of cardiovascular death, myocardial infarction, stent thrombosis, or target vessel revascularization at 1 year (4.5% vs 7.3%, relative risk [RR] 0.59, 95% CI: 0.28–1.24; $P = .16$). However, several patients randomly assigned to IVUS did not receive it, and many patients assigned to the angiography-guided arm had IVUS guidance. In a per protocol analysis according to IVUS usage, IVUS guidance resulted in a significantly larger minimum lumen diameter (2.58 vs 2.51 mm, $P = .04$) and significantly reduced the rate of major adverse cardiac events (4.0% vs 8.1%;, RR 0.48, 95% CI 0.23–0.99; $P = .048$).[48]

Meta-Analysis
Meta-analysis performed in the BMS era reported that IVUS-guided stenting significantly decreased 6-month angiographic restenosis and the rate of target vessel revascularization.[4] A subsequent meta-analysis that included 7 randomized studies also showed that IVUS-guided BMS implantation reduced angiographic restenosis, repeat revascularization, and major adverse cardiac effects, with a neutral effect on death and myocardial infarction.[5]

Recently, Ahn and colleagues[6] performed a comprehensive meta-analysis to evaluate the clinical impact of IVUS-guided PCI with DES compared with conventional angiography-guided PCI. A total of 26,503 patients were included from 3 randomized and 14 observational studies. In this analysis, IVUS-guided PCI was associated with a significantly reduced risk of target lesion revascularization (odds ratio [OR] 0.81, 95% CI 0.66–1.00, $P = .046$) and myocardial infarction (OR 0.57, 95% CI 0.44–0.75, $P<.001$), as well as a lower risk of death (OR 0.61, 95% CI 0.48–0.79, $P<.001$), stent thrombosis (OR 0.59, 95% CI 0.47–0.75, P<.001), and the composite of the death, myocardial infarction, or repeated revascularization (OR 0.74, 95% CI 0.64–0.85, P<.001) over a follow-up period of 12 months to 4 years.

Guidelines for Intravascular Ultrasound Use

Table 3 summarizes the current society guidelines for IVUS use. Both guidelines advocated use of IVUS for stent optimization and for evaluation of the mechanism of stent failure.[49,50]

LIMITATIONS OF INTRAVASCULAR ULTRASOUND

Physical limitations of IVUS are the characteristic signal dropout behind calcium, which prohibits the visualization of deep vessel structures when calcium is present. The physical size of ultrasound catheters (currently ≈1.0 mm) constitutes an important limitation in imaging severe stenoses (which impede catheter crossing) and small vessels. In the latter case, the introduction of the catheter may cause dilatation of the vessel (Dotter effect) and may affect accurate measurements. Several artifacts such as ring-down, geometric distortion, or nonuniform rotational distortion may adversely affect ultrasound images. Compared with angiography-guided PCI, the use of IVUS-guided PCI was associated with implantation of longer and more stents.[6] IVUS guidance is associated with a higher risk of periprocedural myocardial infarction, although IVUS is associated with more stents implanted, longer stenting, and larger-diameter stents.[51] The cost of the IVUS catheter

Table 3
Summary of ACCF/AHA/SCAI and ESC/EACTS guidelines for IVUS

Guidelines	Class of Recommendation	Level of Evidence
2011 ACCF/AHA/SCAI Guideline	**IIa**	
	IVUS is reasonable for the assessment of angiographically indeterminate left main coronary artery disease	B
	IVUS and coronary angiography are reasonable 4–6 wk and 1 y after cardiac transplantation to exclude donor coronary artery disease, detect rapidly progressive cardiac allograft vasculopathy, and provide prognostic information	B
	IVUS is reasonable to determine the mechanism of stent restenosis	C
	IIb	
	IVUS may be reasonable for the assessment of nonleft main coronary arteries with angiographically intermediate coronary stenoses (50%–70% diameter stenosis)	B
	IVUS may be considered for guidance of coronary stent implantation, particularly in cases of left main coronary artery stenting	B
	IVUS may be reasonable to determine the mechanism of stent thrombosis	C
	III	
	IVUS for routine lesion assessment is not recommended when revascularization with PCI or CABG is not being contemplated	C
2014 ESC/EACTS Guideline	**IIa**	
	IVUS in selected patients to optimize stent implantation	B
	IVUS to assess severity and optimize treatment of unprotected left main lesions	B
	IVUS to assess mechanisms of stent failure (restenosis and stent thrombosis)	C

Abbreviation: CABG, coronary artery bypass graft.

may be a major barrier to the implementation of IVUS evaluation in everyday practice.

SUMMARY

The primary rationale for the use of IVUS during PCI is to plan interventional strategy and optimize stent deployment. The use of IVUS to identify which lesions should be treated is problematic: recent data suggest that an MLA ≤ 2.4 mm^2 is the optimal cutoff to predict functional significance by FFR, although IVUS-derived MLA alone cannot replace noninvasive or invasive functional assessment. Stent optimization by IVUS includes the evaluation of stent expansion, apposition, lesion coverage, and the presence or absence of stent edge dissection. Observational studies suggest that IVUS guidance during DES implantation reduces the risk of major adverse cardiac events, particularly in the setting of unprotected left main PCI. The as-treated analysis of the long-lesion RESET trial reported that the use of IVUS guidance resulted in significantly larger MSA and a lower risk of major adverse cardiac events compared with angiographic guidance alone. IVUS is a key imaging tool during PCI, particular in the complex patient and lesion cohorts.

REFERENCES

1. Mintz GS, Nissen SE, Anderson WD, et al. American College of Cardiology Clinical Expert Consensus Document on Standards for Acquisition, Measurement and Reporting of Intravascular Ultrasound Studies (IVUS). A report of the American College of Cardiology Task Force on Clinical Expert Consensus Documents. J Am Coll Cardiol 2001;37:1478–92.

2. Mintz GS. Clinical utility of intravascular imaging and physiology in coronary artery disease. J Am Coll Cardiol 2014;64:207–22.

3. Mintz GS, Weissman NJ. Intravascular ultrasound in the drug-eluting stent era. J Am Coll Cardiol 2006; 48:421–9.

4. Casella G, Klauss V, Ottani F, et al. Impact of intravascular ultrasound-guided stenting on long-term clinical outcome: a meta-analysis of available studies comparing intravascular ultrasound-guided and angiographically guided stenting. Catheter Cardiovasc Interv 2003;59:314–21.

5. Parise H, Maehara A, Stone GW, et al. Meta-analysis of randomized studies comparing intravascular ultrasound versus angiographic guidance of percutaneous coronary intervention in pre-drug-eluting stent era. Am J Cardiol 2011;107:374–82.

6. Ahn JM, Kang SJ, Yoon SH, et al. Meta-analysis of outcomes after intravascular ultrasound-guided

7. McDaniel MC, Eshtehardi P, Sawaya FJ, et al. Contemporary clinical applications of coronary intravascular ultrasound. JACC Cardiovasc Interv 2011;4:1155–67.

8. Kang SJ, Lee JY, Ahn JM, et al. Validation of intravascular ultrasound-derived parameters with fractional flow reserve for assessment of coronary stenosis severity. Circ Cardiovasc Interv 2011;4: 65–71.

9. Nishioka T, Amanullah AM, Luo H, et al. Clinical validation of intravascular ultrasound imaging for assessment of coronary stenosis severity: comparison with stress myocardial perfusion imaging. J Am Coll Cardiol 1999;33:1870–8.

10. Briguori C, Anzuini A, Airoldi F, et al. Intravascular ultrasound criteria for the assessment of the functional significance of intermediate coronary artery stenoses and comparison with fractional flow reserve. Am J Cardiol 2001;87:136–41.

11. Takagi A, Tsurumi Y, Ishii Y, et al. Clinical potential of intravascular ultrasound for physiological assessment of coronary stenosis: relationship between quantitative ultrasound tomography and pressure-derived fractional flow reserve. Circulation 1999; 100:250–5.

12. Abizaid A, Mintz GS, Pichard AD, et al. Clinical, intravascular ultrasound, and quantitative angiographic determinants of the coronary flow reserve before and after percutaneous transluminal coronary angioplasty. Am J Cardiol 1998;82:423–8.

13. Kang SJ, Ahn JM, Song H, et al. Usefulness of minimal luminal coronary area determined by intravascular ultrasound to predict functional significance in stable and unstable angina pectoris. Am J Cardiol 2012;109:947–53.

14. Ben-Dor I, Torguson R, Deksissa T, et al. Intravascular ultrasound lumen area parameters for assessment of physiological ischemia by fractional flow reserve in intermediate coronary artery stenosis. Cardiovasc Revasc Med 2012;13:177–82.

15. Koo BK, Yang HM, Doh JH, et al. Optimal intravascular ultrasound criteria and their accuracy for defining the functional significance of intermediate coronary stenoses of different locations. JACC Cardiovasc Interv 2011;4:803–11.

16. Gonzalo N, Escaned J, Alfonso F, et al. Morphometric assessment of coronary stenosis relevance with optical coherence tomography: a comparison with fractional flow reserve and intravascular ultrasound. J Am Coll Cardiol 2012;59:1080–9.

17. Nakamura S, Colombo A, Gaglione A, et al. Intracoronary ultrasound observations during stent implantation. Circulation 1994;89:2026–34.

18. Brodie BR, Cooper C, Jones M, et al. Postdilatation clinical comparative study I. Is adjunctive balloon postdilatation necessary after coronary stent deployment? Final results from the POSTIT trial. Catheter Cardiovasc Interv 2003;59:184–92.

19. de Ribamar Costa J Jr, Mintz GS, Carlier SG, et al. Intravascular ultrasound assessment of drug-eluting stent expansion. Am Heart J 2007;153: 297–303.

20. Fujii K, Carlier SG, Mintz GS, et al. Stent underexpansion and residual reference segment stenosis are related to stent thrombosis after sirolimus-eluting stent implantation: an intravascular ultrasound study. J Am Coll Cardiol 2005;45:995–8.

21. Okabe T, Mintz GS, Buch AN, et al. Intravascular ultrasound parameters associated with stent thrombosis after drug-eluting stent deployment. Am J Cardiol 2007;100:615–20.

22. Sonoda S, Morino Y, Ako J, et al. Impact of final stent dimensions on long-term results following sirolimus-eluting stent implantation: serial intravascular ultrasound analysis from the SIRIUS trial. J Am Coll Cardiol 2004;43:1959–63.

23. Hong MK, Mintz GS, Lee CW, et al. Intravascular ultrasound predictors of angiographic restenosis after sirolimus-eluting stent implantation. Eur Heart J 2006;27:1305–10.

24. Doi H, Maehara A, Mintz GS, et al. Impact of postintervention minimal stent area on 9-month follow-up patency of paclitaxel-eluting stents: an integrated intravascular ultrasound analysis from the TAXUS IV, V, and VI and TAXUS ATLAS workhorse, long lesion, and direct stent trials. JACC Cardiovasc Interv 2009;2:1269–75.

25. Shimada Y, Honda Y, Hongo Y, et al. Sirolimus-eluting stent implantation in small coronary arteries: predictors of long-term stent patency and neointimal hyperplasia. Circulation 2005;112:U800.

26. Song HG, Kang SJ, Ahn JM, et al. Intravascular ultrasound assessment of optimal stent area to prevent in-stent restenosis after zotarolimus-, everolimus-, and sirolimus-eluting stent implantation. Catheter Cardiovasc Interv 2014;83:873–8.

27. Liu X, Doi H, Maehara A, et al. A volumetric intravascular ultrasound comparison of early drug-eluting stent thrombosis versus restenosis. JACC Cardiovasc Interv 2009;2:428–34.

28. Sakurai R, Ako J, Morino Y, et al. Predictors of edge stenosis following sirolimus-eluting stent deployment (a quantitative intravascular ultrasound analysis from the SIRIUS trial). Am J Cardiol 2005;96:1251–3.

29. Suh J, Park DW, Lee JY, et al. The relationship and threshold of stent length with regard to risk of stent thrombosis after drug-eluting stent implantation. JACC Cardiovasc Interv 2010;3:383–9.

30. Ahn JM, Han S, Park YK, et al. Differential prognostic effect of intravascular ultrasound use according to implanted stent length. Am J Cardiol 2013;111:829–35.

31. Choi SY, Witzenbichler B, Maehara A, et al. Intravascular ultrasound findings of early stent thrombosis after primary percutaneous intervention in acute myocardial infarction: a Harmonizing Outcomes with Revascularization and Stents in Acute Myocardial Infarction (HORIZONS-AMI) substudy. Circ Cardiovasc Interv 2011;4:239–47.

32. Hong MK, Park SW, Lee NH, et al. Long-term outcomes of minor dissection at the edge of stents detected with intravascular ultrasound. Am J Cardiol 2000;86:791–5. a9.

33. Liu X, Tsujita K, Maehara A, et al. Intravascular ultrasound assessment of the incidence and predictors of edge dissections after drug-eluting stent implantation. JACC Cardiovasc Interv 2009;2:997–1004.

34. Yoon HJ, Hur SH. Optimization of stent deployment by intravascular ultrasound. Korean J Intern Med 2012;27:30–8.

35. Hong MK, Mintz GS, Lee CW, et al. Late stent malapposition after drug-eluting stent implantation: an intravascular ultrasound analysis with long-term follow-up. Circulation 2006;113:414–9.

36. Tanabe K, Serruys PW, Degertekin M, et al. Incomplete stent apposition after implantation of paclitaxel-eluting stents or bare metal stents: insights from the randomized TAXUS II trial. Circulation 2005;111:900–5.

37. Guo N, Maehara A, Mintz GS, et al. Incidence, mechanisms, predictors, and clinical impact of acute and late stent malapposition after primary intervention in patients with acute myocardial infarction: an intravascular ultrasound substudy of the Harmonizing Outcomes with Revascularization and Stents in Acute Myocardial Infarction (HORIZONS-AMI) trial. Circulation 2010;122: 1077–84.

38. Cook S, Wenaweser P, Togni M, et al. Incomplete stent apposition and very late stent thrombosis after drug-eluting stent implantation. Circulation 2007;115:2426–34.

39. Steinberg DH, Mintz GS, Mandinov L, et al. Long-term impact of routinely detected early and late incomplete stent apposition: an integrated intravascular ultrasound analysis of the TAXUS IV, V, and VI and TAXUS ATLAS workhorse, long lesion, and direct stent studies. JACC Cardiovasc Interv 2010;3:486–94.

40. Roy P, Waksman R. Intravascular ultrasound guidance in drug-eluting stent deployment. Minerva Cardioangiol 2008;56:67–77.

41. Hur SH, Kang SJ, Kim YH, et al. Impact of intravascular ultrasound-guided percutaneous coronary intervention on long-term clinical outcomes in a real world population. Catheter Cardiovasc Interv 2013;81:407–16.

42. Witzenbichler B, Maehara A, Weisz G, et al. Relationship between intravascular ultrasound guidance and clinical outcomes after drug-eluting stents: the assessment of dual antiplatelet therapy with drug-eluting stents (ADAPT-DES) study. Circulation 2014;129:463–70.

43. Kim SH, Kim YH, Kang SJ, et al. Long-term outcomes of intravascular ultrasound-guided stenting in coronary bifurcation lesions. Am J Cardiol 2010;106:612–8.

44. Hahn JY, Chun WJ, Kim JH, et al. Predictors and outcomes of side branch occlusion after main vessel stenting in coronary bifurcation lesions: results from the COBIS II Registry (Coronary Bifurcation Stenting). J Am Coll Cardiol 2013;62:1654–9.

45. de la Torre Hernandez JM, Baz Alonso JA, Gomez Hospital JA, et al. Clinical impact of intravascular ultrasound guidance in drug-eluting stent implantation for unprotected left main coronary disease: pooled analysis at the patient-level of 4 registries. JACC Cardiovasc Interv 2014;7:244–54.

46. Jakabcin J, Spacek R, Bystron M, et al. Long-term health outcome and mortality evaluation after invasive coronary treatment using drug eluting stents with or without the IVUS guidance. Randomized control trial. HOME DES IVUS. Catheter Cardiovasc Interv 2010;75:578–83.

47. Chieffo A, Latib A, Caussin C, et al. A prospective, randomized trial of intravascular-ultrasound guided compared to angiography guided stent implantation in complex coronary lesions: the AVIO trial. Am Heart J 2013;165:65–72.

48. Kim JS, Kang TS, Mintz GS, et al. Randomized comparison of clinical outcomes between intravascular ultrasound and angiography-guided drug-eluting stent implantation for long coronary artery stenoses. JACC Cardiovasc Interv 2013;6:369–76.

49. Windecker S, Kolh P, Alfonso F, et al. 2014 ESC/EACTS Guidelines on myocardial revascularization. EuroIntervention 2015;10:1024–94.

50. Levine GN, Bates ER, Blankenship JC, et al. 2011 ACCF/AHA/SCAI Guideline for Percutaneous Coronary Intervention: a report of the American College of Cardiology Foundation/American Heart Association Task Force on Practice Guidelines and the Society for Cardiovascular Angiography and Interventions. Circulation 2011;124:e574–651.

51. Park KW, Kang SH, Yang HM, et al. Impact of intravascular ultrasound guidance in routine percutaneous coronary intervention for conventional lesions: data from the EXCELLENT trial. Int J Cardiol 2013;167:721–6.

Moving?

Make sure your subscription moves with you!

To notify us of your new address, find your **Clinics Account Number** (located on your mailing label above your name), and contact customer service at:

Email: journalscustomerservice-usa@elsevier.com

800-654-2452 (subscribers in the U.S. & Canada)
314-447-8871 (subscribers outside of the U.S. & Canada)

Fax number: 314-447-8029

Elsevier Health Sciences Division
Subscription Customer Service
3251 Riverport Lane
Maryland Heights, MO 63043

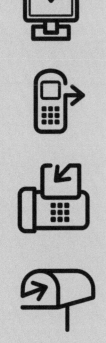

ELSEVIER

Printed and bound by CPI Group (UK) Ltd, Croydon, CR0 4YY

03/10/2024

01040379-0017